Building the Medical Record

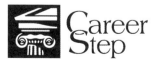
Career Step

Medical Transcription Program
3rd Edition

Career Step, LLC
Phone: 801.489.9393
Toll-Free: 800.246.7837
Fax: 801.491.6645
careerstep.com

This text companion contains a snapshot of the online program content converted to a printed format. Please note that the online training program is constantly changing and improving and is always the source of the most up-to-date information.

Table of Contents

Unit 1
Introduction

Building the Medical Record – Introduction

Learning Objective

The purpose of this module is to educate the student on how to build the medical record. Specifically, the module will cover report types, report components, formatting rules, and effective use of resources. The physical exam and laboratory data report components will be studied in detail in this module. Finally, this module will cover medical ethics and confidentiality as they relate to healthcare documentation in medical transcription.

Like most things in life, it is easier to transcribe a medical report if you fully understand the type of medical report you will be working on and its respective components. It makes sense, doesn't it? If someone asked you to bake a cake, first you would want to know what kind of cake he or she had in mind: a sheet cake, a cheesecake, an angel food cake, a fruit cake (probably not, but one never knows), or maybe a pound cake? Next, you'd need to acquire the ingredients necessary to bring that cake to fruition, or "fruit-ition" in the case of that dreaded fruit cake. You certainly couldn't be expected to make a German chocolate cake with walnut icing if you didn't know the ingredients. Once you learned the components 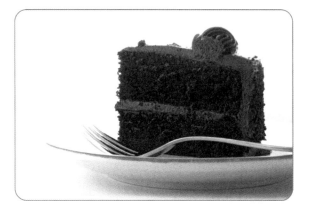 (ingredients) of the cake—off to the store! By now, in addition to the craving for dessert you have, you are probably wondering how all of this translates into building the medical record. Think of the medical report as the cake and the report components as the ingredients. When the components are brought together, they form the medical report itself.

While it is certainly possible to transcribe medical reports without fully understanding them, doing so would not likely yield an accurate and an efficiently produced document. Imagine skipping two or three ingredients in your German chocolate cake. It may look like a cake, but it certainly wouldn't taste right. Have you ever uttered the words "It tastes like it's missing something"? So, too, would be the case if components were absent from the medical record. In this module we will cover the various types of medical record reports, and then deconstruct the report to fully understand all the components of it. We will also illustrate formatting of reports and how to use resources effectively and efficiently to produce accurate medical reports. We will begin with work types. (And now that I am hungry for cake, I think I'll go grab a handful of almonds...)

Unit 2
Work Types

Work Types – Introduction

The medical record, whether inpatient or outpatient, is the *who*, *what*, *where*, *when* and *how* of patient care. In general, a patient's medical record is made up of some or all of the following types of reports.

Report Type	Classification	Sample Headings
Clinic Note	Medical Clinic Multispecialty Clinic	Subjective Objective Assessment Plan
Progress Note	Medical Clinic Multispecialty Clinic Acute Care/ Hospital	Subjective/History of Present Illness Objective/Physical Examination Assessment Plan
Letter	Medical Clinic Multispecialty Clinic Acute Care/ Hospital	Does not typically use headings except the typical greeting and salutation.
Emergency Room	Acute Care/ Hospital	Chief Complaint History of Present Illness Past Medical History Allergies Current Medications Review of Systems Physical Examination Laboratory Findings Assessment and Plan Discharge Instructions
History and Physical	Acute Care/ Hospital	Chief Complaint History Of Present Illness Past Medical History Allergies Current Medications Social History Family History Review of Systems Physical Examination Laboratory Data Admitting Diagnosis or Assessment Plan

Consultation	Multispecialty Clinic Acute Care/ Hospital	Referring Physician Reason for Consultation Chief Complaint History of Present Illness Past Medical History Physical Examination Laboratory Data Assessment Recommendations
Operative Note	Acute Care/ Hospital	Preoperative Diagnosis Postoperative Diagnosis Operation Performed Surgeon Anesthesia Estimated Blood Loss Complications Indications for Operation Findings Description of Operation
Procedure Note	Medical Clinic Multispecialty Clinic Acute Care/ Hospital	Preoperative Diagnosis Postoperative Diagnosis Procedure Performed Surgeon Indications for Procedure Findings Description of Procedure
Discharge Summary	Acute Care/ Hospital	Admitting Diagnosis History of Present Illness Past Medical History Social History Family History Review of Systems Physical Examination Laboratory Data Hospital Course Discharge Diagnoses Discharge Medications Disposition
Radiology	Medical Clinic Multispecialty Clinic Acute Care/ Hospital	Clinical History Report Type Impression
Pathology	Multispecialty Clinic Acute Care/ Hospital	Clinical History Gross Examination Microscopic Examination Diagnoses

I. TRUE/FALSE.
Mark the following true or false.

1. A clinic note generally contains the headings of Chief Complaint and Hospital Course.
   ○ true
   ○ false

2. If the doctor does not dictate all headings, the transcriptionist is free to insert the ones he or she sees fit.
   ○ true
   ○ false

3. The four main headings one might see in a clinic note are Subjective, Objective, Assessment, and Plan.
   ○ true
   ○ false

4. A letter done in the transcription setting typically uses headings and/or subheadings.
   ○ true
   ○ false

5. Report components are always the same in medical reports.
   ○ true
   ○ false

6. The term *medical record* is applied to both inpatient and outpatient types of reports.
   ○ true
   ○ false

7. The heading of Family History is only found on the history and physical report.
   ○ true
   ○ false

8. One of the headings a transcriptionist can expect to encounter on a radiology report is Gross Examination.
   ○ true
   ○ false

9. In simple terms, the *who, what, when, where*, and *how* of a patient comprises the medical record.

   ○ true
   ○ false

10. Both operative notes and procedure notes usually have a preoperative diagnosis as well as a postoperative diagnosis dictated.

    ○ true
    ○ false

Clinic Notes and Acute Care Work Types

Typically, the work type is tied to the kind of facility rendering care. If, for example, you transcribe for an outpatient facility (medical clinic, radiology clinic, multispecialty clinic), you would generally transcribe clinic notes, letters, radiology reports, progress notes, and some procedure notes. If, however, you transcribe for an inpatient facility (hospital), you would most likely spend your days (or nights) transcribing history and physicals, progress notes, consultations, operative notes, procedure notes, discharge summaries, ER Reports, and some radiology reports. Of note, pathology reports are often transcribed by MTs who specialize in pathology. To that end, they are not included in this breakdown. In a very general and broad way, we often classify transcription into two levels—Clinic Notes and Acute Care. In fact, the practicum modules in this training program are broken down into clinic notes, basic acute care, and advanced acute care modules. (But we are putting the cart before the horse—whoa Nelly, back to work types!) Let's break it down by the work types you will likely be exposed to most.

Clinic Note

Medical clinics and a variety of multispecialty clinics use the SOAP (pronounced soap) formatting for reports. This is a quite common method of formatting routine or problem-oriented physician visits.

> **SOAP** stands for **S**ubjective, **O**bjective, **A**ssessment, and **P**lan.

History and Physical (H&P)

If you work on an acute care account you will likely transcribe your fair share of these reports. H&Ps are generated upon patient admittance to the hospital and are used for reference throughout the hospital stay. An H&Ps primary function is to provide background information on new patients and outline what is planned for the hospital stay.

Consultation

A consultation is done when a physician other than the attending physician (or the attending service) examines and/or performs tests on a patient. It is not uncommon for a patient admitted to the hospital to undergo several consultations from more than one specialist.

Operative Note

An operative report (or procedure note) is generated upon completion of any type of surgical procedure. These are required for same-day surgeries and admitted patients.

Discharge Summary

Just as a patient admitted to the hospital has an admission history and physical, they are also required to have a discharge summary. A discharge summary contains all the information found in the history and physical, plus the hospital course and discharge plans. This, as the name implies, is a summary of all that happened before the patient was discharged.

Emergency Room (ER) Reports

Emergency departments provide urgent care to patients. Patients treated in emergency departments and discharged the same day are considered hospital outpatients. The increased use of emergency room services for more routine care has resulted in a large volume of healthcare documentation for ER outpatients.

Radiology Report

A radiology report is any type of an x-ray examination. These include, but are certainly not limited to, chest x-rays, backs, hips, arms, feet, toes, fingers, skull, CT and MRI examinations, upper GIs, ultrasounds, bone age tests, etc. They typically follow a relatively simple format.

Now let's take a closer look at some sample reports from the various work types. This exposure will help you put the information you have learned in this unit so far into context.

Clinic Note

To review, medical clinics and a variety of multispecialty clinics use clinic notes in the SOAP format for medical reports. This is a quite common method of formatting routine or problem-oriented physician visits. When you go to your family physician, a clinic note is generated. When you visit your dermatologist for your annual skin care screen (You do this, right? Especially those of you in our sunshine states?), a clinic note is generated. It is likely that you will transcribe a lot of clinic notes in your career as an MT, and it is definite that you will transcribe them in this training program!

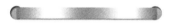

Medical Record

SUBJECTIVE: Status post removal of multiple large lesions. The patient returns for recheck of excision site and pathology results.

OBJECTIVE: Everything is healing well. She is having a little bit of separation or scabbing in the area of the most significant tension portion of the flap on her thigh; however, it should still heal well. Everything is intact. Everything is healing well. She has good circulation.

ASSESSMENT: Status post removal of multiple large lesions, healing well.

PLAN: We will exchange her Steri-Strips in all areas. She will need to continue to change these Steri-Strips or Hypafix tape. She was given a good supply of both hypoallergenic Steri-Strips and Hypafix along with Mastisol. The larger bottle of Mastisol, not the small bottle, will be given to her and will be charged separately as alternative medical supplies.

Other than that, she is healing well, and the pathology was discussed with her. Specifically, I spent considerable time discussing the dysplastic nevus, which was removed. However, the surgical margins were clear, so no further excision will be done at this point.

SUBJECTIVE: This 50-year-old white male, established patient at this facility, hurt his shoulder about a month ago and also has an intermittent right sciatica. He has been using two 800 mg Motrin tablets 3 times a day without relief. He quit his alcohol use just before Christmas.

OBJECTIVE: Vital signs show blood pressure 137/83, weight 152, temperature 98.3, and pulse 69. There is tenderness of the left posterior shoulder, made worse by elevation. There is also faint tenderness of the neck. There is no palpable lumbosacral tenderness. Straight leg raises are negative. Strength is adequate in all extremities.

ASSESSMENT

1. Left shoulder pain.
2. Sciatica.

PLAN

1. Discontinue ibuprofen.
2. Naprosyn 500 mg 1 tablet twice a day with food as needed for back pain. Patient was counseled to take one of these twice a day, and if he does not see some improvement within 2 weeks to return to see me. He was also counseled not to use this longer than 2 weeks.
3. The patient was offered to take blood work today to check his kidneys and liver, although he refused this due to another commitment. He has to get back to work.
4. Return if symptoms persist. Otherwise, schedule followup appointment in 2 weeks.

History and Physical

When a patient is to be admitted to the hospital, a history and physical examination is performed. The document typically includes the patient's past medical history, and often the family and social history, and outlines any medications the patient is taking. The physician completes a detailed review of systems, performs a comprehensive physical exam, and usually orders tests, x-rays, and lab work related to the patient's condition or symptoms (for example, an electrocardiogram [EKG], chest x-ray, comprehensive blood panel, etc.). An assessment of medical problems is typically included, as is a plan for management and treatment. If the projected hospitalization includes plans for a surgical procedure, this report may also be called a "Preoperative History and Physical."

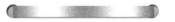

CHIEF COMPLAINT: Left inguinal hernia.

HISTORY OF PRESENT ILLNESS: This established patient is a 59-year-old male who has a 3-month history of a tender left inguinal hernia. The patient first noticed this problem last fall. The patient describes the pain as being constant but mild. The hernia is reducible. The patient reports the hernia is also warm; however, the patient denies any changes in bowel or bladder habits, any blood in the urine or stool, or any nausea or vomiting. Patient also denies any change in stool caliber.

PAST MEDICAL HISTORY: The patient has hypercholesterolemia, as well as tinnitus. Tinnitus was diagnosed last year.

PAST SURGICAL HISTORY: The patient has had a sinus operation 15 years ago.

ALLERGIES: THE PATIENT HAS NO KNOWN MEDICAL ALLERGIES.

CURRENT MEDICATIONS: The patient takes gemfibrozil 600 mg p.o. b.i.d., ibuprofen 800 mg p.o. t.i.d. p.r.n., and simvastatin 20 mg q.h.s.

SOCIAL HISTORY: The patient has never been a smoker. The patient denies alcohol use and other illicit drug use as well. The patient has been divorced for 3 years and currently lives by himself. He has 3 children, all sons.

FAMILY HISTORY: Negative for coronary artery disease, strokes, cancer, and diabetes.

REVIEW OF SYSTEMS: The patient reports he has had approximately a 10% weight loss in the past couple of months; however, this weight loss has been permissible. Otherwise, review of systems is noncontributory. The patient denies chest pain, palpitations, or syncope. Denies shortness of breath or wheezing. Denies nausea or vomiting. Denies headaches or syncope.

PHYSICAL EXAMINATION: General: This is a 59-year-old white male, awake, alert, and oriented x3, very pleasant to talk to, who is sitting comfortably in a chair in no acute distress. Vital signs: Temperature 97.0, heart rate 75, respiratory rate 20, blood pressure 156/101. Patient has a 98% saturation on room air. HEENT: Head is normocephalic, atraumatic. Pupils are equally round and reactive to light and accommodation. Extraocular muscles are intact. There is no icterus. Mucous membranes are moist. Neck: Supple with good range of motion. Trachea is midline. There was no JVD or lymphadenopathy present. Chest: The lungs are clear to auscultation bilaterally. Heart: Regular rate and rhythm without murmur. Abdomen: Soft, nontender, and nondistended. Bowel sounds are present. Extremities: Warm. There is no clubbing, cyanosis, or edema noted. GU exam: Patient has a readily apparent left inguinal hernia. The sac will pulse or bulge with any increase in intra-abdominal pressure. The hernia is reducible. It is also tender to palpation. Rectal exam: The patient has normal sphincter tone. There is stool present in the vault; however, there is no gross blood present on examination. Prostate is enlarged but soft.

ASSESSMENT: The patient is a 59-year-old white male who is here for a preoperative history and physical. The patient is otherwise healthy.

PLAN: The patient is scheduled to have a left inguinal hernia repair done tomorrow.

HISTORY OF PRESENT ILLNESS: This is a 78-year-old white male, established patient, with a past medical history significant for coronary artery disease with 3-vessel CABG and atrial flutter who was admitted for medical cardioversion using propafenone.

The patient developed an atrial flutter after undergoing a CABG procedure 8–9 years ago. Previously the patient was DC cardioverted for the atrial flutter. The patient did respond to the DC cardioversion and returned to a normal sinus rhythm for 3 weeks. However, the patient eventually reverted back to an atrial flutter rhythm after being cardioverted. The patient then underwent an ablation therapy for the atrial flutter but the procedure was unsuccessful.

The patient is currently asymptomatic at this time. However, the patient's symptoms are usually confined to lethargy during episodes of regular heartbeat that he can notice. The patient denies any paroxysmal nocturnal dyspnea, any orthopnea, or any decrease in exercise tolerance.

PAST MEDICAL HISTORY

1. Three-vessel coronary artery bypass graft.
2. Bilateral carotid endarterectomies.
3. Left femoral-popliteal bypass.
4. Atrial flutter refractory to sotalol, DC cardioversion, and ablation therapy.
5. Diabetes mellitus.
6. Hyperlipidemia.
7. Hypertension.

FAMILY HISTORY

1. Mother died of Hodgkin's disease.
2. Father died at age 94 due to natural causes.
3. No siblings who had any history of heart disease.
4. No family history of hypertension or diabetes mellitus type 2.

SOCIAL HISTORY: The patient has a 120-pack-year history for smoking. The patient is a social drinker and he denies any illicit drug use.

MEDICATIONS: Admission medications include Coumadin 3 mg per day, simvastatin 30 mg at night, potassium chloride 10 mEq every other day, ranitidine 150 mg at night, nitroglycerin sublingual p.r.n. for chest pain, metoprolol 50 mg b.i.d., felodipine 5 mg daily, glipizide 2.5 mg every morning, digoxin 0.125 mg daily, and nitroglycerin patch 0.2 mg remove at night.

The patient had an echocardiogram showing an ejection fraction of 65% and concentric LVH.

REVIEW OF SYSTEMS: General: The patient denies any fevers, chills, and excessive weight gain or weight loss. The patient denies any recent history of trauma or headaches. Eyes: The patient denies any discharge from the eyes, itchiness of the eyes, or double vision. Ears: The patient denies any discharge from the ears or tinnitus. Nose: The patient denies any rhinorrhea or difficulty breathing. Throat: The patient denies any thyromegaly or difficulty swallowing. Cardiovascular: The patient denies any paroxysmal nocturnal dyspnea, orthopnea, or decrease in exercise tolerance. Respiratory: The patient denies any history of TB, pneumonia, or shortness of breath. Gastrointestinal: The patient denies any blood in stools, any diarrhea, constipation, nausea, or vomiting. Endocrine: The patient denies any excessive weight gain or weight loss, any excessive heat or cold intolerance. Neurological: The patient denies any seizures, numbness, tingling, or memory loss. Renal: The patient denies any polyuria, dysuria, or difficulty urinating.

PHYSICAL EXAMINATION: Vital signs showed a pulse of 54, blood pressure 123/68, temperature 97.5, and a respiratory rate of 14. In general, the patient is alert and oriented with no acute distress, and is a well-developed, well-nourished male. HEENT revealed a patient who has a normocephalic, atraumatic head. Extraocular muscles are intact. Pupils were equal, round, and reactive to light bilaterally. No evidence of jugular venous pulsations. No thyromegaly, no scleral icterus, and no evidence of lymphadenopathy. Cardiovascular examination revealed S1 and S2 to be present with a regularly irregularly heartbeat and distant heart sounds. No murmurs, gallops, or rubs were appreciated. Lungs showed clear to auscultation bilaterally with good air entry bilaterally. No accessory muscles were being used. No rales, rhonchi, or wheezing was appreciated. Abdominal examination showed no tenderness, no distention, no masses, and positive bowel sounds. Extremities revealed no clubbing, cyanosis, or edema. Pedal pulses were present and there was evidence of scars secondary to the fem-popliteal procedure. Neurological examination showed cranial nerves 2–12 to be grossly intact, and no focal deficits.

ASSESSMENT/PLAN: Atrial flutter. The patient will be converted using propafenone. Cardiology will start this medication and titrate appropriately. We will restart the patient on his home medications. We will obtain serial EKGs in the morning. The patient will also get blood results of PT, INR, PTT, basic metabolic panel, magnesium, and phosphate, and Cardiology will continue to follow this patient.

Consultation

To review, a consultation is done when a physician other than the attending physician (or the attending service) examines and/or performs tests on a patient. It is not uncommon for a patient admitted to the hospital to undergo several consultations from more than one specialist. Consultations often include a REFERRING PHYSICIAN and a REASON FOR CONSULTATION heading.

Medical Record

REASON FOR CONSULTATION: Right lower lobe lung nodule.

HISTORY OF PRESENT ILLNESS: Patient is an established 63-year-old white male with a 2-year history of squamous cell T4 N0 M0 pharyngeal tumor treated with chemotherapy and radiation therapy, which was complicated by post radiation dysphagia resulting in permanent J-tube placement.

Last week he had a chest x-ray, which revealed a new right lower lobe 3 cm lung nodule, which was confirmed by CT scan that revealed a peripheral lung nodule. Patient stated his weight has been stable and he feels well.

A CT-guided needle biopsy is scheduled by ENT. We were asked to evaluate to see if another option is to do a bronchoscopy for this nodule.

ALLERGIES: None.

MEDICATIONS: He takes occasional Tylenol.

SOCIAL HISTORY: Quit tobacco 1–1/2 years ago. He smoked 2 packs per day for 40 years. Moderate alcohol use. No drug use. He was a painter for 40 years without airway protection.

FAMILY HISTORY: He has a grandmother with breast cancer.

REVIEW OF SYSTEMS: No fevers, chills, or night sweats. Has gained weight. No headaches. HEENT: No visual or auditory changes. Positive sinus problems. Positive dysphagia since radiation. Had a barium swallow which revealed that his pharynx would never close appropriately for eating; therefore, he is fed through a permanent J-tube. Neck: Positive pain secondary to radiation. Chest: No chest pain, palpitations, edema, or orthopnea. Lungs: Had PFTs last week. He does have some dyspnea on exertion and occasional cough. GI: No hematochezia, melena, nausea, or vomiting. No abdominal pain. He has a J-tube in place. GU: Negative. Musculoskeletal: Negative. Skin: Negative.

PHYSICAL EXAMINATION: General: Vitals per electronic note. He is a thin white male who appears to be in no acute distress. Neck has hard skin changes secondary to radiation. No lymphadenopathy. Very limited range of motion. HEENT: Tympanic membranes were normal. Nasal mucosa had some clear rhinorrhea and pale mucosa. Unable to fully open mouth, therefore unable to evaluate the posterior pharynx, but did have a normal-appearing mucosa from what could be seen. Heart: Regular rate and rhythm. No murmurs, rubs, or gallops. Lungs are clear to auscultation bilaterally. No wheezes, rhonchi, or rales. No retractions noted.

LABORATORY DATA: Pulmonary function tests showed a normal FEV1 of 4.21, which is 121% of predicted. FEV1/FVC of 80. Lung volumes and diffusion were normal.

ASSESSMENT/PLAN: Right lower lobe peripheral lung nodule. Suspect metastatic squamous cell carcinoma. We will get a needle biopsy, which is already scheduled for next week by his ENT. We will present his case to determine further course of action after diagnosis obtained from CT-guided needle biopsy.

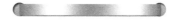

Medical Record

HISTORY OF PRESENT ILLNESS: The patient is an 11-year-old white female who suffered a bad biking accident today, with multiple abrasions, and embedded foreign body into the multiple abrasions on her face, torso, and hands

The only injury, which is gaping open, is a very extensive avulsion laceration of her lower lip, with severe trauma to her lower incisor dental area with some fractures involving the base of the teeth. They did make an appointment for today, to see their dentist for their tooth-related problem; however, she does have a very complex laceration extending entirely through her orbicularis oris muscle, with some avulsion of the buccal gingival area, which will require some flap closure of the gingiva. This will also be pertinent for survival of the teeth, by maintaining adequate blood supply to the area. She presents today upon referral from her primary care physician for consultation and potential repair.

PAST MEDICAL HISTORY: The patient states that she is otherwise healthy with no other medical problems.

PAST SURGICAL HISTORY: Denies any significant past surgical history.

ALLERGIES: No known allergies.

MEDICATIONS: None.

SOCIAL HISTORY: Nonsmoker, nondrinker.

FAMILY HISTORY: Negative for hemophilia. Both parents are alive and well and so are all her siblings with no chronic illnesses or conditions.

REVIEW OF SYSTEMS: As noted above, otherwise negative.

PHYSICAL EXAM
GENERAL: Well-developed, well-nourished afebrile patient.
NEUROLOGIC: Normal affect and mood. Alert and oriented x3.
EYES: Pupils are equally round and reactive to light. Extraocular movements are intact.
HEAD/EARS/NOSE/MOUTH/OROPHARYNX: Traumatic-appearing face. Ears, nose, and oropharynx are without abnormality. The head, face, lips, and mouth are as noted in HPI with lacerations and abrasions.
NECK: Supple, full range of motion. No adenopathy. No thyroid gross abnormality.
LUNGS: Clear to auscultation and percussion. Normal respiratory effect.
HEART: Regular rate and rhythm, without murmur.
CARDIOVASCULAR: No gross edema, or significant varicosities.
ABDOMEN: Soft, nontender, nondistended. No hepatosplenomegaly or masses. Normal bowel sounds.
EXTREMITIES: Within normal limits.
MUSCULOSKELETAL: Generally unremarkable. Normal gait. No asymmetry. Normal range of motion.
LYMPHATIC: No adenopathy, neck and axilla.
SKIN: No visual or palpable gross irregularities on areas examined. She has no tendon injuries.

ASSESSMENT/PLAN: Biking accident today, with multiple abrasions, embedded foreign body into the multiple abrasions on her face, torso, and hands, and a gaping extensive avulsion laceration of her lower lip, with severe trauma to her lower incisor dental area, and with some fractures involving the base of the teeth.

PROCEDURE: Debridement, as well as possible, was done of all the abrasions and embedded foreign bodies throughout the areas. Topical anesthetic was placed so that the patient could shower at home and further clean the areas. She will continue to put antibiotic ointment on these areas as well. Surgical intervention will be acutely required for the avulsion of the buccal gingiva on her lower lip and repair of the large laceration extending through the orbicularis oris muscle of the lip.

PLAN: We will take the patient to the operating room immediately for repairs to be done on an outpatient basis. The risks, complications, and alternatives of the procedures have been explained to the patient and her mother and all their questions answered. The patient's mother signed the consent to proceed with surgery.

Operative Note

Each time an operation or procedure is performed, an operative report or procedure note is generated. This document lists important information, such as the preoperative and postoperative diagnoses, type of operation, reason for operation, description of operation, and findings.

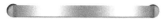

Medical Record

PREOPERATIVE DIAGNOSIS: Left ureteral stricture.

POSTOPERATIVE DIAGNOSIS: Left ureteral stricture.

OPERATION PERFORMED: Left ureteral stent change under anesthesia.

DRAINS: 7 French hydrophilic microvasive 24-cm left ureteral stent.

INDICATIONS: The patient is a 49-year-old white male who has left ureteral stricture secondary to colon cancer and radiation. He has frequent calcification of his stents and needs them changed every 2 months. He presents for change.

DESCRIPTION OF PROCEDURE: Consent was obtained. The patient was given an IV sedative, placed on the operating table in the dorsal lithotomy position, and prepped and draped in the usual sterile fashion. The urethra was anesthetized with 2% Anestacon. The 21 French cystoscopic sheath and 4 oblique lens were placed into the bladder under direct vision without difficulty. The left ureteral stent was identified and removed using alligator forceps. The 21 French cystoscopic sheath and 4 oblique lens were then placed into the bladder under direct vision again. Using the glide wire the left ureteral orifice was cannulated. Plain films showed good position of the tip of the glide wire in the left renal pelvis. The stent was then passed over the guide wire and pushed in place using a pusher and the guide wire removed. There was one full turn left in the bladder. Plain film confirmed good position of the stent. The bladder was emptied, and the scope was removed. The patient was taken out of the lithotomy position, moved under his own power to a gurney, and transported to the recovery room in stable condition. There were no complications, and the patient tolerated this procedure well.

Medical Record

PREOPERATIVE DIAGNOSIS: Nevus of the midback and nevus of the left lower back.

POSTOPERATIVE DIAGNOSIS: Nevus of the midback and nevus of the left lower back.

PREOPERATIVE SIZE: Midback 0.8 x 0.6 cm; left lower back 0.6 x 0.4 cm.

POSTOPERATIVE DEFECT SIZE: Midback 3.0 cm; left lower back 0.6 cm.

PROCEDURE: Excision of nevus, mid-lower back with complex layer closure; punch biopsy of nevus, left lower back.

DESCRIPTION OF PROCEDURE: The relevant risks and aspects, as well as the rights of refusal were explained to the patient. The informed consent was obtained and placed on the chart.

The patient was brought to the operating suite, and the two areas on the back were prepped and draped in the usual sterile manner. A fusiform shape was drawn around the lesion on the mid-lower back. The area was then infiltrated with anesthetic. A #15 scalpel was used to excise down to the level of subcutaneous fat. The tissue was removed and sent to pathology. The edges were undermined with blunt scissor dissection. Hemostasis was maintained with electrocautery. The subcutaneous layer was closed with 3 sutures of 4-0 Vicryl. The cutaneous layer was reapproximated with a running suture of 4-0 nylon. A 6-mm punch biopsy was used to remove the nevus of the left lower back. The subcutaneous layer was reapproximated with one suture of 4-0 Vicryl. The cutaneous layer was closed with 3 sutures of 4-0 nylon.

ANESTHESIA: 5 cc of lidocaine with 1:100,000 epinephrine.

ESTIMATED BLOOD LOSS: Minimal.

COMPLICATIONS: None.

DISPOSITION: The patient was alert and oriented times 3 post procedure and tolerated the procedure well. He was given both verbal and written wound care instructions. He is to follow up on Friday at 8:30 a.m. for suture removal.

Discharge Summary

A discharge summary is the report generated when a patient is being discharged from an inpatient hospital admission. The patient's name is listed, as well as the admission date and discharge date, although this information has been stripped from most of the files you will deal with in this training program in an effort to protect patient confidentiality. A brief history explaining why the patient was admitted is presented here, as well as a generalized description, although a detailed description of the patient's hospital course (what was done and why during the hospital stay) is preferred. A final diagnosis is included and a listing of any and all procedures performed during the patient's hospital stay.

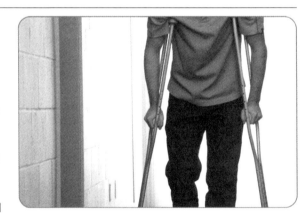

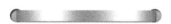

Medical Record

CHIEF COMPLAINT: Monocular diplopia and blurry vision, OD, secondary to cataract.

HISTORY OF PRESENT ILLNESS: Monocular diplopia and blurry vision, OD, secondary to cataract.

PAST MEDICAL HISTORY: Positive for rheumatoid arthritis, hypothyroidism, and chronic open angle glaucoma.

PAST SURGICAL HISTORY: Status post benign breast mass excision, total abdominal hysterectomy.

SOCIAL HISTORY: She denies use of tobacco and alcohol.

MEDICATIONS: Timoptic b.i.d. OU, levothyroxine 0.075 mg daily, quinine 325 mg p.r.n. cramps, amitriptyline 25 mg at bedtime, Plaquenil 200 mg b.i.d., estrogen 0.625 mg daily.

ALLERGIES: She has a questionable allergy to oral antibiotics; however, she does not know which antibiotic.

REVIEW OF SYSTEMS: Noncontributory.

PHYSICAL EXAMINATION: Other than ocular, physical exam is within normal limits. Ocular exam: 20/40+, OU. She glares to 20/50 in both eyes. Tonometry by applanation at 0900, 14 and 16 mmHg respectively. The pupils are equal. Anterior segment exam is normal in both eyes. Dilated fundus exam: Lens reveals she has 2+ nuclear sclerosis with cortical changes in both eyes, somewhat more severe in the right than the left. Cup-to-disc: 0.4 with temporal sloping, OU. Disc is normal, OU. Macula normal, OU; periphery normal, OU.

DISCHARGE DIAGNOSES

1. Cataract, right eye.
2. Rheumatoid arthritis.
3. Hypothyroidism.
4. Chronic open angle glaucoma.

PROCEDURE: Phacoemulsification with posterior chamber IOL, right eye.

DISCHARGE MEDICATIONS

1. Tylenol with codeine 1-2 q.4-6 hours p.r.n. pain.
2. Diamox Sequels 500 mg p.o. q.1600 and at bedtime.

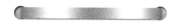

Medical Record

DIAGNOSES

1. Fracture of the inferior ramus of the pubis on the right.
2. Heme positive stool.
3. Anemia.
4. Dementia.
5. Weight loss.

HISTORY OF PRESENT ILLNESS: The patient is a 71-year-old male who had fallen somehow the night before admission. He had landed sitting, facing his bed, and he complained of his right leg hurting and not being able to walk. He usually could walk and exercise and was quite vigorous. He was seen last year for organic brain syndrome, but had no physical disability. He was on Motrin for occasional arthritic pain. He has a long history of weight loss and was to be admitted for barium enema electively the day after his presentation to the emergency room. He denied pain but was unable to stand.

PAST MEDICAL HISTORY: His weight has gone from 97 pounds to 92 pounds in 3 months. He had a urinary tract infection which showed no growth but was symptomatic. He has anemia with a hemoglobin of 11 noted 3 months ago. He has a history of organic brain syndrome with paranoia. He is status post left cerebral artery aneurysm, for which he had surgery. Following this he has had his organic brain syndrome. He is status post TURP for urinary retention and elevated PSA.

MEDICATIONS: Motrin p.r.n.

ALLERGIES: No known allergies.

SOCIAL HISTORY: He lives with his wife, and his children live next door.

REVIEW OF SYSTEMS: He had no complaints other than inability to stand.

PHYSICAL EXAMINATION: Older man who was sitting up with his right hip flexed at 45 degrees, externally rotated, and his knee flexed 45 degrees. He was moaning with exploration, but that is his usual. Temperature 96.9, pulse 78, respirations 18, blood pressure 150/62. Exam was essentially negative. Rectal was heme positive with normal prostate. His right leg was as described above. He was able to straighten the leg but could not rotate it to neutral. He could not weightbear. He was tender over the anterior ramus of the pubis on the right. Otherwise his extremities were normal except for being wasted.

LABORATORY DATA: Hemoglobin 9.3, hematocrit 28, with 17.6 lymphs and a white count of 5.2. Chemistries were normal except for an albumin of 3.3. X-ray showed a crack in the inferior ramus on the right.

HOSPITAL COURSE: The patient was admitted and put on bedrest. X-rays were reviewed with the radiologist, who agreed that there was a fracture of the inferior ramus of the pubis. The patient was discussed with orthopedics, who felt that gradual increase in weightbearing with a walker was best for him. He was seen by dietary who felt that he was at 84% of ideal body weight. He was given Enrich supplement. He did not have a large amount of pain. He had his barium enema as had been previously scheduled. He showed no gross pathology, but it was a limited study. After the barium enema the patient was able to weightbear and appeared happy and with minimal pain. He was discharged to home.

PROCEDURES: Barium enema, walker education.

DISCHARGE INSTRUCTIONS: He was set up for a followup appointment. He was to take an iron rich diet. After his followup it will be decided whether or not he needs to have iron supplements.

DISCHARGE MEDICATIONS: Motrin 400 mg p.o. t.i.d. three months supply and a walker were dispensed.

CONDITION AT DISCHARGE: Improved.

Emergency Room

Because patients treated in the emergency room are treated for such a wide variety of problems, it would be impossible to give you an example of everything you could expect to encounter. However, the format for emergency room report is basically the same everywhere and for all types of problems, unless they are extremely severe, in which case the patient will be admitted.

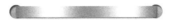

Medical Record

CHIEF COMPLAINT: Thrown from horse with loss of consciousness.

HISTORY OF PRESENT ILLNESS: This is an apparently 16-year-old female who was riding a horse today and was thrown, striking her head. She apparently was knocked out for 1 to 2 minutes, and after that awoke, being somewhat combative and confused. She was brought by ambulance here to the emergency department.

PHYSICAL EXAMINATION: This 16-year-old girl is in no acute distress, although she is intermittently somewhat confused and minimally combative. She has blood and fluid coming out of her left ear. No distal neurologic deficit is noted on gross exam. Cranial nerves 2–12 are grossly intact as well. Deep tendon reflexes 2+ and equal bilaterally. No focal or lateralized deficits are demonstrable. Chest is clear. Breath sounds are bilaterally equal without rales, rhonchi, or wheezes. No rib tenderness is noted. Her abdomen is soft, nontender, without guarding, masses, or organomegaly. Bowel sounds are active.

LABORATORY: Noncontrast CAT scan reveals pneumocranium on the left, with some edema of the left temporal lobe.

DIAGNOSIS: Cerebral contusion with basilar skull fracture.

ER TREATMENT: The patient's status was discussed with the attending physician. We elected to admit her to the ICU unit and monitor her for 24 hours.

Medical Record

CHIEF COMPLAINT: Altercation with facial injury.

HISTORY OF PRESENT ILLNESS: This is a 46-year-old lady who complains that she was hit in the face with a fist. This occurred at 2:15 a.m. She was hit multiple times. She had no loss of consciousness. She says that the right side of her nose and upper lip are numb. She has mild soreness of the left shoulder and left thigh.

PAST MEDICAL HISTORY: Negative.

MEDICATIONS: None.

ALLERGIES: None known.

IMMUNIZATION STATUS: Not current.

PHYSICAL EXAMINATION: Vital signs: Temperature 98, pulse 88, respirations 20, blood pressure 120/76. This is a well-developed, well-nourished Caucasian female who is alert and oriented times 3. Head, eyes, ears, nose, and throat exam is significant for tenderness at the left mandibular angle. There is some ecchymosis present here as well and pain with attempted motion of the jaw. The right mandibular condyle is somewhat tender as well. There is some right infraorbital tenderness, swelling, and anesthesia. Pupils are equal, round, reactive to light. There is no entrapment of upper gaze. In fact, the extraocular movements are intact in all directions. There is minimal amount of nasal tenderness, which is not clinically significant. Head, eyes, ears, nose, and throat exam is otherwise negative with hemotympanum. There is mild tenderness and swelling of the right posterior parietal scalp. There is also some mild tenderness of the left deltoid laterally and the lateral hips. Range of motion is quite good with both joints, that is, left shoulder and left hip. Distal neurovascular exam is intact. There is no neck, chest, back, or pelvis tenderness. Heart has regular rate and rhythm without murmurs. Lungs are clear to auscultation bilaterally. Abdomen is soft and nontender.

DIAGNOSTIC STUDIES: X-ray studies of the mandible and face reveal fracture of the left side of the mandible through the base of the coronoid process and most probably through the neck as well, along the base of the neck. It appears nondisplaced. Facial x-rays reveal an air/fluid level in the right maxillary sinus. No distinct fracture line is identified. Serum pregnancy test is negative.

ER TREATMENT: A CT was done to determine the exact site of maxillary sinus fracture and the exact nature of the mandibular fracture. The patient is turned over at this time, 8:20 in the evening, to the attending service, who will obtain the results of the CT and coordinate the patient's further care.

Radiology

The radiology report documents the type of x-ray that was performed, what the radiologist saw when viewing the film(s), and the final impression of the x-ray by the radiologist. The radiologist rarely takes the x-rays. However, he/she always interprets them and generates a report that is sent back to the ordering physician. Many clinics and specialty practices have their own radiology technicians who perform standard x-rays in-office and then the physician (not a radiologist) reviews the films and interprets them. Many types of x-rays, such as CT scans, MRIs, upper GI series, OB ultrasounds, nuclear scans, and more, are performed in the hospital setting simply due to the cost of owning the equipment to perform such radiologic procedures. In these circumstances the films are reviewed by the radiologist and a report is generated back to the ordering physician.

Medical Record

CLINICAL HISTORY: A 52-year-old patient status post thoracentesis, rule out pneumothorax.

PORTABLE CHEST X-RAY: There is no evidence of pneumothorax. There is no opacification of the right lower hemothorax compatible with effusion.

IMPRESSION: No evidence of pneumothorax.

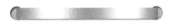

Medical Record

CLINICAL HISTORY: Not dictated.

ABDOMINAL ULTRASOUND: Extremely limited exam was performed in correlation with the recently performed MRI. Patient did not present with a full bladder, and therefore the pelvis was not evaluated in detail. Again noted is the hydronephrosis of the right kidney with an ill-defined, hypoechoic density that extends caudal to the right kidney into the pelvis, best seen with the patient in the left lateral decubitus position. On reviewing the MRI, this mass correlates with the location of the right iliopsoas muscle.

IMPRESSION

1. Right flank mass, which extends caudal to the right kidney into the pelvis, which is poorly defined but can be identified by ultrasound, and therefore ultrasound can be used for localization for needle biopsy.
2. Repeat ultrasound with full bladder may be warranted.

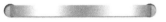

Medical Record

CLINICAL HISTORY: Large right frontal mass on CT scan in patient with left upper lobe lung lesion, question metastasis versus primary tumor.

MRI OF THE BRAIN

PROCEDURE: Sagittal T1 weighted images were obtained through the brain, followed by proton density and T2 weighted images in the axial plane. These were followed by axial T1 weighted images pre and post Magnevist injection.

FINDINGS: There are multiple enhancing lesions noted in both hemispheres of the brain. The largest lesion is in the right frontoparietal region near the gray/white junction. This lesion demonstrates extensive white matter edema with mass effect upon the frontal horn of the right lateral ventricle and mild right-to-left shift. Two smaller lesions are noted, one in the posterior left parietal region and a second in the anterior left temporal region. These lesions also enhance with gadolinium.

IMPRESSION: Multiple enhancing lesions in both cerebral hemispheres, consistent with metastatic disease. The largest of these lesions in the right frontoparietal region has extensive surrounding white matter edema with mass effect and mild right-to-left shift.

Unit 3
Report Components

Report Components – Introduction

Now that we have discussed the type of reports you will be exposed to, it makes sense to jump into report components. As you will recall from our cake analogy earlier, the report components are the "ingredients" needed to make the cake, or in this case, the medical report itself. (Hmm, now I am hungry for cake again!) If we break down the medical record we can inspect each component and put it back together again with a better understanding of how it goes together.

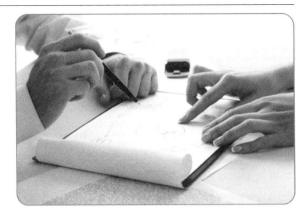

While all report types do not follow one specific template of headings (wouldn't that make life easier?), there are general headings associated with each work type. This will make more sense as we work through the examples in this unit. Let's begin with clinic notes.

Clinic Note Components

In general, clinic notes are broken down into SOAP format, and are often even referred to as such. SOAP is an acronym for the first letter of each heading in the report:

S – SUBJECTIVE
O – OBJECTIVE
A – ASSESSMENT
P – PLAN

Some accounts use a format that includes the same information as the SOAP format, but the headings are different, and some use a combination of SOAP and other headings. Alternative headings include, but are not limited to:

HISTORY
PHYSICAL EXAMINATION
DIAGNOSIS
RECOMMENDATIONS

When transcribing clinic notes you will find that some dictators will not even say the entire heading but will recite only the letter instead. For example, the dictator might say "S colon" for the subjective heading. Depending on the account instructions, you might expand this out to SUBJECTIVE: or you might simply transcribe this as S:. It is also the case that many dictators use the basic SOAP format, but they never dictate any headings at all. In this case account instructions will often dictate whether you add headings or transcribe the report verbatim (with no headings). If you are to add the appropriate headings when required, it is essential to know what each heading is actually describing. Let's break them down.

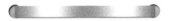

Medical Record

SUBJECTIVE: A narrative of the patient's own description of his/her complaints. This would include any past history or review of systems, allergies, or medication lists that are provided.

OBJECTIVE: The description of the physician's findings on observation and examination, any physical signs, and laboratory testing or diagnostic studies, such as x-rays.

ASSESSMENT: How the physician interprets the findings (both subjective and objective). In other words, this is the physician's opinion, impression, assessment, or diagnosis.

PLAN: For treatment and followup. This includes any medication regimen, instruction (such as elevation or cleansing), suggested education, and followup instruction.

I. MULTIPLE CHOICE.
Choose the best answer.

1. The A in the SOAP formula stands for *Assessment*, which indicates _____.
   - ○ Treatment and followup, including medication regimen, instruction, suggested education, and followup instruction.
   - ○ How the physician interprets the findings; an opinion, impression, assessment, or diagnosis
   - ○ A narrative of the patient's own description of his/her compaints: a past history, review of systems, allergies, or medication lists
   - ○ The description of the physician's findings on observation and examination, any physical signs, and laboratory testing or diagnostic studies, such as x-rays.

2. The P in the SOAP formula stands for *Plan*, which indicates _____.
   - ○ Treatment and followup, including medication regimen, instruction, suggested education, and followup instruction
   - ○ How the physician interprets the findings; an opinion, impression, assessment, or diagnosis
   - ○ A narrative of the patient's own description of his/her compaints: a past history, review of systems, allergies, or medication lists
   - ○ The description of the physician's findings on observation and examination, any physical signs, and laboratory testing or diagnostic studies, such as x-rays

3. The S in the SOAP formula stands for *Subjective*, which indicates _____.

   ○ Treatment and followup, including medication regimen, instruction, suggested education, and followup instruction

   ○ How the physician interprets the findings; an opinion, impression, assessment, or diagnosis

   ○ A narrative of the patient's own description of his/her compaints: a past history, review of systems, allergies, or medication lists

   ○ The description of the physician's findings on observation and examination, any physical signs, and laboratory testing or diagnostic studies, such as x-rays

4. The O in the SOAP formula stands for *Objective*, which indictes _____.

   ○ Treatment and followup, including medication regimen, instruction, suggested education, and followup instruction

   ○ How the physician interprets the findings; an opinion, impression, assessment, or diagnosis

   ○ A narrative of the patient's own description of his/her compaints: a past history, review of systems, allergies, or medication lists

   ○ The description of the physician's findings on observation and examination, any physical signs, and laboratory testing or diagnostic studies, such as x-rays

Standard Acute Care Components

Acute care reports are the documentation for patient care rendered in an inpatient setting. The standard acute care reports (H&P, discharge summary, consults, and even ER reports) will include information such as the reason the patient is being cared for, the patient's history, the current condition, evaluation, diagnostic evaluation, treatment, assessment of condition, and plan going forward. This information will typically fall under one of the headings listed below, although there are other headings or report components used in acute care reports. Again, a thorough understanding of what information falls under each component will help you put together a more accurate document—which will effectively help you become a high-quality MT. You can have your cake and eat it, too (nudge, nudge, wink, wink)!

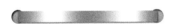

Medical Record

CHIEF COMPLAINT: The chief complaint, as the name implies, is the principal or main concern, issue, or reason for being seen. In a consultation report this might be referred to as REASON FOR CONSULTATION, but they mean the same thing. The information following this heading tells us why the patient is being seen, for example: a sprained ankle, heart palpitations, a motor vehicle collision, a peanut in the nose, etc.

HISTORY: The history information in a medical record is frequently broken down into a number of history categories (each generally with their own headings). The content under history headings gives us vital information regarding what treatment has been received in the past, medication history, pertinent family history, and even social history. You can surely imagine how historical information might be used to assess, treat, and diagnose a patient. For example, if a patient comes in with what could feasibly be either indigestion or chest pain, and this patient has a strong family history of congestive heart failure and myocardial infarction, a cardiac workup might be the first evaluation planned.

PAST MEDICAL HISTORY: This is where the past illnesses, diseases, and conditions are listed. This information can be presented in paragraph format or in a list.

SURGICAL HISTORY: This heading will hold information regarding a patient's past surgical history, frequently with dates included.

FAMILY HISTORY: The information under this heading includes information regarding family history of coronary artery disease, strokes, cancer, and diabetes. This will also frequently list whether family members and siblings are living or deceased.

SOCIAL HISTORY: This heading often holds information with regard to marital status, children or no children, employment status and occupational history, hobbies, military service, living arrangements, family structure/dynamics, smoking history, and alcohol use history (sometimes dictated as ETOH).

MEDICATIONS: This heading, as you might suspect, lists medications the patient is or was taking. Alternate medications headings include things like: CURRENT MEDICATIONS, MEDICATIONS LIST, or even MEDICATIONS ON ADMISSION. Sometimes this information is presented in a paragraph and other times in a list. There is much acceptable variation to how drug terminology information is presented.

ALLERGIES: It is very important to document any allergic reactions a patient might have had to medications (or things like latex) to avoid administration of such medications in the future. In fact, many accounts will require any allergy statements BE PRESENTED IN ALL CAPS. A phrase common to the allergy heading is NO KNOWN DRUG ALLERGY. Frequently the allergen is listed with a description of the reaction it evokes.

REVIEW OF SYSTEMS: The review of systems, when fully utilized, is a fairly comprehensive overview of symptoms by body system. These are subjective findings (unlike the physical exam which relates objective findings). Systems commonly covered in the ROS include general/ constitutional, skin, eyes/ears/nose/mouth/throat, cardiovascular, respiratory, GI, GU, musculoskeletal, neurologic, and lymphatic. While these subheadings are not used all the time, they are the most common systems referenced in the ROS.

PHYSICAL EXAMINATION: The physical exam is the examination of the body for signs of disease or changes. The PE can be presented in paragraph format with subheadings left justified or with subheadings embedded throughout the paragraph. Account instructions will typically decide how the information is presented. While the headings may change in a given PE, the exam usually starts at the head and ends with the extremities. The physical exam headings typically include: vital signs, general appearance, HEENT, neck, lungs, heart, abdomen, genitalia, musculoskeletal, neurologic, skin, and extremities. We will take a much closer look at the physical examination in a later unit.

DIAGNOSTIC STUDIES: Information in the diagnostic studies headings typically includes laboratory data, x-ray, or other diagnostic testing. We will take a much closer look at laboratory data in a later unit, including types of lab values and normal ranges.

HOSPITAL COURSE: Evaluation and treatment rendered in the hospital is presented under this heading. In an ER report this might be referred to as ER TREATMENT.

DIAGNOSES/ASSESSMENT: As the name implies, the information under this heading includes the cause or nature of the condition or reason for being seen. These findings are frequently presented in a list format. It is generally preferred to not use abbreviations under the diagnoses heading. For example, if a dictator states "DIAGNOSIS: GERD," this would be expanded out to DIAGNOSIS: Gastroesophageal reflux disease.

PLAN: This heading holds information regarding future treatment and followup. In a discharge summary, the plan might be referred to as DISCHARGE INSTRUCTIONS.

I. FILL IN THE BLANK.
Using the word/word parts in the box, fill in the blanks.

1. This category is often broken down into several more detailed categories. _____

2. In the _____ section, the doctor notes that John is an unmarried college student who does not smoke or drink.

3. The section that indicates evaluation and treatment rendered in a hospital is under the heading _____.

4. _____ is the section that gives a comprehensive overview of symptoms by body system.

5. John comes in complaining of stomach pain. This is an example of the _____.

6. The section is where the body is examined for signs of disease or changes. _____

7. John has a history of stomach ulcers. This would be indicated under _____.

8. The _____ section includes information that John is not currently taking any prescribed medicine.

9. The section that holds information regarding future treatment and followup is _____.

10. Information regarding John's past surgery would be indicated under _____.

Word Box
Allergies
Social History
Family History
Diagnosis/Assessment
History
Surgical History
Plan
Medications
Past Medical History
Diagnostic Studies
Physical Examination
Chief Complaint
Review of Systems
Hospital course

11. The heading labeled _____ includes the cause or

    nature of the condition or reason for being seen.

12. In the _____ section, it is indicated that John's

    mother has a history of acid reflux problems.

13. The _____ section typically includes lab data, e-

    ray, or other testing.

14. This section indicates that John has NO KNOWN DRUG

    ALLERGY. _____

Operative Note Components

Operative reports and procedure notes do not follow the same standard format as most other acute care reports. To review, an operative report (or procedure note) is generated upon completion of any type of surgical procedure. These are required for same day surgeries as well as on admitted patients. The patient's name, medical record number, date of surgery, surgeon, and place of surgery are all listed on the report, but for our purposes (and to protect patient confidentiality) this information has been removed.

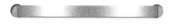

Medical Record

PREOPERATIVE DIAGNOSIS: A preoperative diagnosis is listed to show the probable diagnosis, rule out a diagnosis, or state an unconfirmed diagnosis prior to the procedure.

POSTOPERATIVE DIAGNOSIS: The postoperative diagnosis lists the diagnosis made after the surgery is performed and the surgeon has had the opportunity to explore the diseased body area or organ system thoroughly to pinpoint the problem.

OPERATIONS: This is a very important part of the operative report—it lists all of the surgical procedures (in order of priority) that were performed on the patient during this particular operation.

SURGEON: The physician who performed the surgery.

ASSISTANT SURGEON(S): Any assistant surgeons who were present and assisted the primary surgeon with the operation(s).

ANESTHESIA: The type of anesthetic used, when applicable.

ESTIMATED BLOOD LOSS: The amount of blood loss during the operation/procedure, when applicable.

INDICATION FOR OPERATION: This gives background information on why an operation is being performed. This also frequently lists the consent statement—acknowledgement of the patient (or patient's caretaker) giving verbal or written consent to the operation and an understanding of possible complications.

PROCEDURE: This is an actual description of what occurred during the surgery. It is a minute-by-minute description of the proceedings of the surgery in the order they occurred, the techniques used, and the equipment and supplies used to carry it out.

FINDINGS: The findings section lists the outcome of the surgery, specifying what was found to be the underlying problem or cause of the surgery.

I. MATCHING.
Match the correct heading to the definition.

1. ____ This is listed to show the probable diagnosis, rule out a diagnosis, or state an unconfirmed diagnosis prior to the procedure.

2. ____ This lists the diagnosis made after the surgery is performed and the surgeon has had the opportunity to explore the disease body area or organ system thoroughly to pinpoint the problem.

3. ____ A listing of all the surgical procedures in order of priority that were performed on the patient.

4. ____ The physician who performed the surgery.

5. ____ Any physicians who were present and assisted the primary physician with the operation.

6. ____ The type of anesthetic used.

7. ____ The amount of blood lost during the procedure.

8. ____ The background information on why an operation is being performed.

9. ____ An actual description of what occurred during the surgery.

10. ____ The listing of the outcome of the surgery, specifying what was found to be the underlying problem or cause of the surgery.

A. Findings
B. Preoperative Diagnosis
C. Indication for operation
D. Operations
E. Surgeon
F. Assistant Surgeon(s)
G. Postoperative Diagnosis
H. Estimated blood loss
I. Anesthesia
J. Procedure

Unit 4
Physical Examination

Physical Examination – Introduction

The Physical Examination, sometimes called Physical Exam or PE, is an objective evaluation and physical assessment of the body's systems. This is not to be confused with the Review of Systems, which is a subjective review of the body's symptoms. Basically, the physician inspects the body, feels the various parts (palpation), listens to sounds produced by tapping (percussion) and sounds without tapping (auscultation).

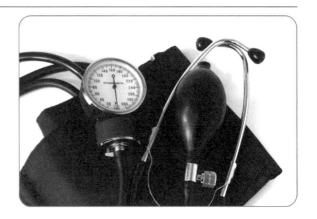

A patient complaining of chest pain might have a longer cardiovascular and/or lung assessment, or perhaps one that is more in depth, during the physical examination. This can occur on an inpatient or outpatient basis, in a clinic or a hospital, so the physical examination is a component that merits an in-depth review as you work your way through this training program.

Elements of the physical exam may include some or all of the following.

- General
    - overall appearance that may include all or some of the following:
        - age
        - race
        - emotional state
        - build of body
        - nutritional state

- Vital Signs
    - temperature
    - blood pressure
    - respiratory rate
    - pulse
    - height
    - weight

- HEENT
    - head
    - eyes
    - ears
    - nose
    - throat

- Neck
- Lungs
- Chest
- Cardiovascular/Heart
- Abdomen
- Genitourinary
- Musculoskeletal/Extremities
- Neurological
- Skin
- Psychiatric

The physical exam is the doctor's objective evaluation of the body and its systems (as opposed to the Review of Systems, which is the *patient's* report of systemic problems). To give you an overview as to how the PE might appear in a medical record, the following is a sample physical examination section of a report:

Physical Examination

PHYSICAL EXAMINATION: When he was first seen in the emergency room he was pale, slightly dyspneic at rest, and otherwise in no acute distress. Vitals: Pulse 120, afebrile, blood pressure 106/40, weight 132 pounds, which is 1 pound less than 1 month ago. Neck: Marked JVD and hepatojugular reflux as before, and again JVD even when standing. Cardiovascular exam: Tachycardia with summation gallop and possible new aortic insufficiency murmur. He still had his very obvious mitral regurgitation. Lungs: Fine basilar rales. Abdomen: Nontender. Liver may be a couple of fingerbreadths below his costal margin but did not percuss large. He did not have any edema. Most significantly, and different from last month, was that his legs demonstrated widespread purpura bilaterally from the midthigh down. Fundi did not reveal any hemorrhage or rough spots. He had no splinter hemorrhages in his extremities.

Sometimes, the subheadings will be *stacked*—that is, in a vertical fashion atop each other and left justified—and other times (as in this example), they will be in paragraph style. You will see the PE done a variety of ways throughout this unit and the entire training program. Dictator preferences, account specifics, and transcription instructions will provide you the direction needed to set this up properly.

Physical Examination Abbreviations

"The patient was AAO until an hour ago when on A&P, some congestion was heard. Family doctor was called, and an EKG was ordered STAT!" Perhaps you've heard those words spoken by a character on one of the many medically themed TV shows airing these days. In reality, these funky sounding words actually have meaning. (You didn't think the writers made them up, did you?)

An abbreviation is simply a shortened form of a word or a phrase that is used in place of the whole. Abbreviations are prevalent in the world of medicine, and you can expect they will be interspersed throughout the physical examination. It is important for you, as a transcriptionist, to have an understanding of what these abbreviations mean. Doctors will often use a shortened form of a word (the abbreviation) to succinctly and quickly convey the medical information they need to have documented in the medical record. Having an understanding of these medical *shortcuts* will assist you greatly in your journey to become a medical transcriptionist.

The next time you are watching a medical show on TV, try to decipher some of the abbreviations you hear. Hearing them and seeing the context in which they are used is a fun way to process and learn this information. Doctor's orders!

In the lessons that follow we will review frequently used abbreviations associated with the physical examination. For the most part, abbreviations have more than one translation or meaning, so it is generally best to consult your references for variations when you are working as an MT. The abbreviations presented here, however, are all relative to the physical exam.

PE Abbreviations – Lesson 1

I. **ENTER ABBREVIATIONS.**
   Enter the abbreviation and what it stands for.

A&P: auscultation and percussion
Subheading: General, Heart/Cardiovascular

   1. _____ (Abbreviation)

   2. _____

BP: blood pressure
Subheading: Vital Signs

   3. _____ (Abbreviation)

   4. _____

CCE: clubbing, cyanosis, or edema
Subheading: Extremities

   5. _____ (Abbreviation)

   6. _____

CNS: central nervous system
Subheading: Neurology

   7. _____ (Abbreviation)

   8. _____

CVA: costovertebral angle
Subheading: Abdomen

   9. _____ (Abbreviation)

   10. _____

RRR: regular rate and rhythm
Subheading: Heart/Cardiovascular

   11. _____ (Abbreviation)

   12. _____

TMs: tympanic membranes
Subheading: HEENT

   13. _____ (Abbreviation)

   14. _____

SOM: serous otitis media
Subheading: HEENT

   15. _____ (Abbreviation)

   16. _____

BUS: Bartholin glands, urethra, and Skene glands
Subheading: OB/GYN

    17. _____ (Abbreviation)

    18. _____

AV: arteriovenous
Subheading: HEENT (AV nicking), Heart/Cardiovascular

    19. _____ (Abbreviation)

    20. _____

II. FILL IN THE BLANK.
Expand the abbreviation for each of the following.

1. CCE_____   2. BUS_____

3. TMs_____   4. A&P_____

5. SOM_____   6. RRR_____

7. BP_____   8. AV_____

9. CNS_____   10. CVA_____

PE Abbreviations – Lesson 2

I. ENTER ABBREVIATIONS.
Enter the abbreviation and what it stands for.

DTRs: deep tendon reflexes
Subheading: Neurological

    1. _____ (Abbreviation)

    2. _____

GI: gastrointestinal
Subheading: GI

    3. _____ (Abbreviation)

    4. _____

EOMs: extraocular movements
Subheading: HEENT

    5. _____ (Abbreviation)

    6. _____

HEENT: head, eyes, ears, nose, throat
Subheading: HEENT

    7. _____ (Abbreviation)

    8. _____

IAC: internal auditory canal
Subheading: HEENT

    9. _____ (Abbreviation)

    10. _____

GU: genitourinary
Subheading: GU

    11. _____ (Abbreviation)

    12. _____

JVD: jugular venous distention
Subheading: Neck

    13. _____ (Abbreviation)

    14. _____

AD: right ear
Subheading: HEENT

    15. _____ (Abbreviation)

    16. _____

AS: left ear
Subheading: HEENT

    17. _____ (Abbreviation)

    18. _____

AU: both ears
Subheading: HEENT

    19. _____ (Abbreviation)

    20. _____

II. MATCHING.
Match the abbreviation with the subheading in which it would be found on a physical exam.
Some answers may be used more than once.

1. ____ IAC
2. ____ JVD
3. ____ AD
4. ____ DTRs
5. ____ AU

A. HEENT
B. Neck
C. Cardiovascular
D. Neurological

PE Abbreviations – Lesson 3

I. ENTER ABBREVIATIONS.
Enter the abbreviation and what it stands for.

JVP: jugular venous pressure
Subheading: Neck

1. _____ (Abbreviation)
2. _____

NAD: no acute distress
Subheading: General

3. _____ (Abbreviation)
4. _____

NCAT: normocephalic, atraumatic
Subheading: HEENT

5. _____ (Abbreviation)
6. _____

OD: right eye
Subheading: HEENT

7. _____ (Abbreviation)
8. _____

OS: left eye
Subheading: HEENT

9. _____ (Abbreviation)
10. _____

OU: both eyes
Subheading: HEENT

11. _____ (Abbreviation)

12. _____

TMJ: temporomandibular joint
Subheading: HEENT

13. _____ (Abbreviation)

14. _____

FHT: fetal heart tone
Subheading: OB/GYN, GU

15. _____ (Abbreviation)

16. _____

PVCs: premature ventricular contractions
Subheading: General, Heart/Cardiovascular

17. _____ (Abbreviation)

18. _____

DTs: delirium tremens
Subheading: Neurology/Mental Status

19. _____ (Abbreviation)

20. _____

II. **FILL IN THE BLANK.**
   Enter the appropriate term to complete the expansion of the abbreviation.

1. FHT – fetal_____ tone

2. NCAT –_____, atraumatic

3. TMJ – temporomandibular _____

4. OD –_____ eye

5. NAD – no acute_____

6. DTs –_____ tremens

7. OU – both_____

8. JVP –_____ venous pressure

9. OS – _____ eye

10. PVCs – premature _____ contractions

PE Abbreviations – Lesson 4

I. **ENTER ABBREVIATIONS.**
    Enter the abbreviation and what it stands for.

PERRLA: pupils equal, round, reactive to light and accommodation
Subheading: HEENT

1. _____ (Abbreviation)

2. _____

PMI: point of maximal impulse
Subheading: Heart/Cardiovascular

3. _____ (Abbreviation)

4. _____

REM: rapid eye movement
Subheading: HEENT

5. _____ (Abbreviation)

6. _____

ROM: range of motion
Subheading: Extremities

7. _____ (Abbreviation)

8. _____

LLQ: left lower quadrant
Subheading: Abdomen

9. _____ (Abbreviation)

10. _____

LUQ: left upper quadrant
Subheading: Abdomen

11. _____ (Abbreviation)

12. _____

RLQ: right lower quadrant
Subheading: Abdomen

13. _____ (Abbreviation)

14. _____

AKA: above-knee amputation
Subheading: Extremities

15. _____ (Abbreviation)

16. _____

BKA: below-knee amputation
Subheading: Extremities

17. _____ (Abbreviation)

18. _____

SOB: shortness of breath
Subheading: Lungs

19. _____ (Abbreviation)

20. _____

II. **FILL IN THE BLANK.**
Enter the appropriate term to complete the expansion of the abbreviation.

1. RLQ – _____ lower quadrant

2. SOB – shortness of_____

3. PERRLA – pupils equal,_____, reactive to light and accommodation

4. BKA – below-knee_____

5. ROM – _____ of motion

6. REM – _____ eye movements

7. PMI – point of_____ impulse

8. AKA – _____-knee amputation

9. LUQ – left_____ quadrant

10. LLQ – left_____ quadrant

Physical Examination Samples

Now that you have an opportunity to see some of the many abbreviations that dictators use in the Physical Exam portion of a report, take a few minutes to glance over the samples below. These are a small representative sampling of sentences, medical terms, and abbreviations an MT can expect to hear when transcribing the PE (Physical Examination) section of a report.

Medical Record

Physical Examination

PHYSICAL EXAMINATION: General: On admission, she was a pleasant, elderly female, conversant, alert, looking comfortable and not acutely ill. Skin exam: Crusting on the left pinna and thickened scaly skin with early decubitus changes on the sacrum and ischial spines, as well as both greater tuberosities. HEENT: Her left TM had a dry perforation. Her right TM was okay. Nose was clear. Pupils were small, but reactive with extraocular motions intact. Fundi could not be seen. She had only a few teeth and some black coating on her tongue from nicotine. Neck: There was no jugular venous distention, no neck masses or adenopathy. Chest: Breasts were quite nodular bilaterally, no dominant masses. Lungs: She had wet crackles at both lung bases one third of the way up bilaterally and fine rales up to one half of the way up. Her respiratory rate on admission was 16. Cardiovascular: Heart exam showed a regular rhythm, normal S1 and S2, no S3 or S4, pulse of 84, blood pressure of 124/56. There was no murmur. She had good pulses in all extremities. Abdomen: Obese with no masses or bruits, no tenderness, no organomegaly. The liver edge was sharp, firm, and nontender. Rectal exam: Poor sphincter tone, no rectal masses, and no stool to guaiac test. Extremities: Trace to 1+ edema to the midshins. The skin on the feet was intact. No clubbing, cyanosis, or edema. Neurological: Vibratory sense absent below the knees and light touch absent below the midfoot. Deep tendon reflexes were absent in the lower extremities. Cranial nerves 2-12 were grossly intact. Gait was normal.

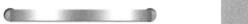

Medical Record

Physical Examination

PHYSICAL EXAMINATION: The patient is a quiet, well-developed, well-nourished young girl in no acute distress, but somewhat uncomfortable. Temperature 97.5 axillary, pulse 76, respirations 12, weight 58 pounds. Ears reveal the right ear is slightly erythematous, slightly bulging, good light reflex and landmarks; left is gray, clear. Eyes show clear sclerae, extraocular muscles intact, pupils equal and reactive to light. Fundi show normal disks and vessels. Nose is crusty and clear with blood-tinged discharge, erythema, and chafing below the nares. On mouth exam, the patient is only able to open slightly, mucous membranes moist. Throat reveals erythema, right tonsillar area much greater than left, but both erythematous without exudates. Neck is supple with large 3–4 cm submandibular nodes, 1–2 cm left submandibular node, tender, not stiff, good anterior occipital movement. Lungs with equal movement without retractions, clear to auscultation without rales, rhonchi, or wheezes. Heart has regular rate and rhythm, S1, S2. Abdomen shows good bowel sounds, soft, nontender, no hepatosplenomegaly or masses. Extremities reveals normal muscle strength. Vascular exam shows 2+ pulses. Neurologic is normal. GU is deferred.

Physical Examination

PHYSICAL EXAMINATION: The patient is an alert x3, well-nourished, 41-year-old Caucasian male. Lesions: The only one seen was ulcer, plantar left foot. Hair: Decreased fullness, male pattern baldness, no scalp lesions. Face is symmetrical. Eyes: Equal, extraocular muscles intact. PERRLA, positive reactivity and positive compensation of the eyes. Nose: Septum midline with a patent air flow, no blockage of the nares. Ears had a positive red reflex, no lesions nor inflammation. Mouth: Positive dentures; gingiva was pink, moist, with no bleeding. Uvula was in the midline. Neck: Supple neck, full range of motion, no pain on range of motion, no carotid bruits, positive +2/4 pulses, no jugular vein distention, no thyromegaly, and trachea was in midline. Lymph nodes: No palpable lymph nodes were noted. Back: Full range of motion and no pain on range of motion. Thorax and lungs: Clear to auscultation bilaterally. No rales, rubs, or crackles were noted with 3 cm distention of the diaphragm on inspiration. Heart: Regular rate and rhythm was noted. No murmurs or gallops, no S3 or S4 heart sounds and +2/4 radial pulses. Abdomen: Obese, soft, no palpable masses or tenderness, bowel sounds times 4+. No hernias. Upper extremity had +3/4 tendon reflexes, +4/5 muscle strength, no pain on range of motion, and full range of motion. Lower extremity exam: +2/4 DP and PT pulses bilaterally, capillary fill time was less than 3 seconds to all digits bilaterally, positive hair growth, no edema; and triphasic Doppler pulse, dorsalis pedis, and posterior tibial pulses bilaterally. Ulcer with hyperkeratotic lesion, sub second metatarsal shaft, left foot, no erythema, no odor, no streaking, and the ulcer measured 1 cm in diameter. Musculoskeletal: The patient had +5/5 muscle strength in all four quadrants, +2/4 Achilles tendon reflex, +2/4 patellar reflex, and amputated toes bilaterally. Neurological: The patient had decreased sharp/dull, but had intact proprioception and vibratory sense with no clonus and no Babinski bilaterally.

I. **MULTIPLE CHOICE.**
   Choose the best answer.

1. In the first medical record example, what part of the exam indicated a dry perforation in the left TM?
   - ◯ Lungs
   - ◯ Neck
   - ◯ Abdomen
   - ◯ HEENT

2. What does HEENT mean?
   - ◯ head, esophagous, eyes, nose, throat
   - ◯ head, eyes, ears, nose, throat
   - ◯ hearing, eyesight, eating habits, nasal function, throat function
   - ◯ head motion, eyesight, ear function, nasal inflamation, throat swelling

3. In the first medical record example, no CCE is present. What is CCE?
   ○ clubbing, cyanosis, or edema
   ○ coughing, cracking, or edema
   ○ clubbing, cracking, or edema
   ○ coughing, cyanosis, or eating disorder

4. In the second medical record example, what does the abbreviation GU indicate?
   ○ gastrointestinal
   ○ genitourinary
   ○ gastrourinary
   ○ genitointestinal

5. In the third medical record example, the doctor indicates positive reactivity and positive compensation of the eyes. This is in reference to what?
   ○ HEENT
   ○ GU
   ○ PERRLA
   ○ DP and PT

6. In the third medical record example, the heart is noted to have a _____.
   ○ RRR- regular rate and rhythm
   ○ IRR- irregular rate and rhythm
   ○ R3- regular rate and rhythm
   ○ RRaR- regular rate and rhythm

Physical Examination Subheadings

As you now know, the Physical Examination (PE) is a summary of the objective findings of the person conducting the actual exam—the examiner/physician. The Physical Exam often consists of subheadings that cover the many body systems observed by the physcian. These subheadings tend to follow a specific format, regardless of who you work for or what account you are assigned. So as you work through these subheadings, keep in mind that the order in which the subheadings are presented is generally the customary way they are dictated in the "real world."

Below is an example of a typical Physical Exam portion of a report in which the subheadings are stacked vertically. On the following pages, we will dissect each of these subheadings so that you become familiar with the content and information contained in each.

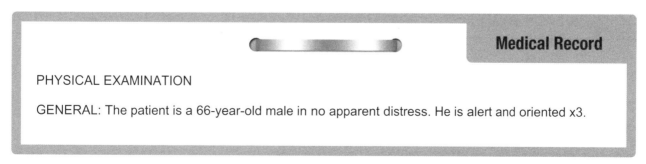

Medical Record

PHYSICAL EXAMINATION

GENERAL: The patient is a 66-year-old male in no apparent distress. He is alert and oriented x3.

VITAL SIGNS: Temperature 97.7, pulse 60, respirations 20, blood pressure 156/82, and O2 saturation 94% on room air.

HEENT: Head is normocephalic. Extraocular muscles are intact. Pupils are equally round and reactive to light and accommodation. Nares are patent. Mouth reveals very poor dentition. Mucous membranes are moist. Posterior pharynx is without lesions or exudate.

NECK: Supple. No JVD. No carotid bruits. No lymphadenopathy.

LUNGS: Clear to auscultation bilaterally.

CARDIOVASCULAR: Regular rate and rhythm but bradycardic. There is an approximate 2/6 to 3/6 systolic murmur heard along the left sternal border. There is mechanical clicking of S2. The patient has a sternal scar present with keloid formation.

ABDOMEN: Obese, soft, nontender, nondistended. Normoactive bowel sounds. No palpable masses.

EXTREMITIES: No clubbing, cyanosis, or edema. Peripheral pulses are +2 in the upper and lower extremities bilaterally.

NEUROLOGIC: Cranial nerves 2-12 are grossly intact. Strength is 5/5 in the upper and lower extremities bilaterally.

PSYCHIATRIC: Affect is flat. Patient denies suicidal or homicidal ideations.

SKIN: The patient's skin is dry and somewhat scaly.

I. TRUE/FALSE.
    Mark the following true or false.

1. The order of the body system subheadings generally follows the same order in the real world.
   ◯ true
   ◯ false

2. JVD, as mentioned under the NECK heading, means jugular venous distention.
   ◯ true
   ◯ false

3. In a physical examination medical record, the HEENT subheading should always be first.
   ◯ true
   ◯ false

4. A note of no CCE is found under the cardiovascular heading.
   ◯ true
   ◯ false

General and Vital Signs

General

The first subheading you will most likely find in the Physical Examination is General. This includes the generalities of the patient's current state. Some of these include appearance, state of alertness, personal hygiene, nutritional status, mood, gait, emotional condition, and even anomalies that can be seen with the naked eye (for example, scars, moles, physical defects).

GENERAL Exam Examples

- *The patient is a 54-year-old Caucasian female who is well-nourished, well-developed, and presently in no acute distress.*
- *The newborn showed an Apgar score of 7 at one minute and 8 at five minutes.*
- *She appears in no acute distress although mildly cushingoid with masked facies.*
- *He is awake and oriented x3 with no orthostatic changes.*
- *The patient is a 15-year-old, healthy appearing teenager who is well-developed though slightly obtunded. She is in no acute distress and is responsive, bright, and alert.*

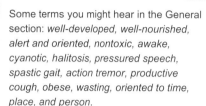

Highlights

Some terms you might hear in the General section: *well-developed, well-nourished, alert and oriented, nontoxic, awake, cyanotic, halitosis, pressured speech, spastic gait, action tremor, productive cough, obese, wasting, oriented to time, place, and person.*

Vital Signs

As you might have guessed, the Vital Signs subheading lists temperature, pulse, respirations, and blood pressure. Sometimes, this information might be given as part of the general examination. These are the quantitative measurements of the patient and are an integral part of the physical examination. Some dictators list the patient's height and weight as well. The temperature might be dictated as Fahrenheit or Celsius. More and more physicians are also expressing patient weight using kilograms (kg), so it is important to properly transcribe what the dictator is saying.

Highlights

Some terms you might hear in the Vital Signs section are: *fever, afebrile, febrile, labored breathing, apical pulse, labile, hypertensive, hypotensive, pansystolic murmur, unobtainable, rectal temperature, pyrexia.*

VITAL SIGNS Exam Examples

- *The patient's temperature is 98.6, afebrile. Her blood pressure is 124/75, pulse 76 and regular.*
- *He is 5 feet 8 inches, weight 215 pounds. Other vital signs not recorded.*
- *Vital signs are stable, but blood pressure was high this morning at 145/90.*

> • *The patient was uncooperative, so blood pressure, pulse, and respiratory rate were unable to be assessed.*
> • *Rectal temperature obtained was 101.3, which is a slight increase over the last 24 hours. Blood pressure and pulse remain stable at 120/80 and 75, respectively.*

I. MULTIPLE CHOICE.
Choose the best answer.

1. Which of the following is NOT an example of a common term in the General section?
   - ○ spastic gait
   - ○ hypotensive
   - ○ obese
   - ○ well-nourished

2. Which of the following is NOT an example of a common term in the Vital Signs section?
   - ○ cyanotic
   - ○ apical pulse
   - ○ labile
   - ○ pyrexia

3. The General subheading typically contains which of the following?
   - ○ temperature, weight, blood pressure, height, etc.
   - ○ description of the head, ears, eyes, nose and throat
   - ○ state of alertness, personal hygiene, appearance, mood, etc.
   - ○ The date, location, and name of the patient

4. Which of the following is an example of what you might find under the Vital Signs subheading?
   - ○ Patient is 54 years old, presenting a productive cough.
   - ○ Muscle tone is good.
   - ○ Abdomen is obese, soft, nontender, nondistended.
   - ○ Patient is 5 feet 6 inches, 175 pounds. Her blood pressure is 124/75.

HEENT

The General and Vital Signs subheadings are typically followed by HEENT, which translates to head, ears, eyes, nose, and throat. If the skin exam is a part of this, it may be referred to as SHEENT. Each of these subtopics are then examined and dictated. For our purposes, we will cover contents under each individual letter in HEENT. Let's break it down!

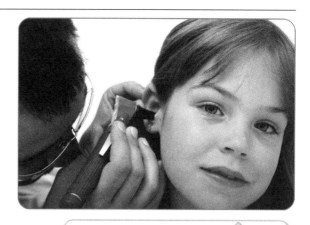

HEAD: Size and shape of the skull, color and texture of skin and hair, facial structure and features, scarring or defects of the head and face, jaw and mouth movement. These are but a few of the many things assessed in exam of the head. Teeth may also be assessed as part of the head exam.

EARS: The tympanic membranes, canals, ossicles, bones, hearing, balance (equilibrium), and physical anomalies are all examined as a part of the ear examination. Expect to hear abbreviations (which were covered in the previous section) such as AD (right ear), AS (left ear), and AU (both ears).

EYES: Examination of the sclerae, corneas, conjunctivae, EOMs (extraocular movements), visual acuity, visual fields, eye chambers, pupils (often transcribed as PERRLA), color vision, fundi, and/or with more in-depth assessment and testing if done by an ophthalmologist.

NOSE: The airway, sinuses, nasal septum, and sense of smell are all considerations in this assessment.

THROAT: If the mouth has not been assessed as part of the head exam, the examiner will often include it as part of the throat assessment. Teeth, lips, gums, tongue, salivary glands, hard and soft palate, uvula, and oral mucosa are all a part of this. Oral cavity inspection is done with the aid of a tongue depressor and light. Pharynx is viewed when the patient says "ahhh" and allows for a closer look. Any lesions, growth, discharge, hemorrhage, or exudates are noted. In addition, the odor of the breath is assessed, as many diseases and conditions are associated with foul or abnormal breath.

Highlights

Some words you might hear in a HEENT examination are:

HEAD: *normocephalic, atraumatic, symmetrical, occiput, alopecia, masked facies, microcephaly, sagittal suture, allergic shiners, facial edema, jaundice.*

EARS: *acoustic meatus, ear canal, eardrum, tympanic membranes, Valsalva maneuver, otitis media, otorrhea, exudate, cerumen, vertigo.*

EYES: *sclerae, dilated pupils, keratitis, globe, ectropion, orbital rim, palpebral fissures, scotoma, accommodation, fundi, intraocular pressure, iritis, anterior segment, corneal ulcer, nystagmus.*

NOSE: *patent nares, rhinorrhea, epistaxis, middle meatus, mucous membrane, boggy turbinates, nasolabial fold, polyps, congestion, sinuses, flattening, hypertrophy.*

THROAT: *tonsillar fossa, gag reflex, tonsillar crypts, erythema, exudates, edentulous, thrush, tongue is midline, cleft palate, phonation.*

HEENT Exam Examples

- *HEAD: Head is atraumatic, normocephalic.*
- *EYES: Pupils are equal, round, and reactive to light and accommodation. EOMs intact.*
- *EARS: Hearing and eardrums are intact.*
- *NOSE: Flattening of the nasolabial fold is present, but otherwise no abnormalities detected.*
- *THROAT: Upon testing of gag reflex, uvula projects upward.*

- *HEENT: Pupils equal, round, and reactive to light. Extraocular movements are full. Nose soft without lesions. Dentition is in adequate condition.*
- *HEENT: Head examination, normocephalic. Positive vitiligo on the right side of the face. Funduscopy normal. No papilledema. No retinal changes. Nose and throat are clear. Ear examination is normal. Throat examination, no signs of infection.*
- *HEENT showed no head trauma. TMs were normal bilaterally with scarring. Pupils were equal, round, and reactive to light. Extraocular motions were intact with no injection. Nares were clear but reddened. The throat was not red, with no exudate. Tongue was tobacco stained. Teeth were in fair repair.*

I. FILL IN THE BLANK.
Enter the correct word in the blank provided.

1. Any scarring or defects of the face would be included under this subheading._____

2. A deviated nasal septum would be indicated under this subheading._____

3. EOM and PERRLA would be examples of information found under this subheading._____

4. An assessment of balance and tympanic membranes would be found under this subheading._____

5. The gag reflex and odor of the breath are assessed under this subheading._____

Neck, Lungs, and Chest

Neck

If not included in the HEENT exam, the neck exam will be dictated separately. Information in this area includes neck mobility, contour, shape, assessment of lymph nodes, tracheal position, distention of neck veins, carotid pulses, limitations on movement, masses, growths, swelling, thyroid gland assessment.

Lungs

In a lung exam, the examiner is listening to breath sounds, lung fields, and the patient is usually seated. A&P are the key methods used in this exam portion and these stand for auscultation (listening) and percussion (tapping). Inhalation and exhalation are performed in order to assess the lungs.

Chest

Sometimes a grouping separate from the lung exam will be performed that concentrates on the chest, breasts, and/or axillae areas. In this case, the size, shape, and symmetry of the breasts is more closely assessed. Breathing movement can also be viewed during this time as part of the overall chest wall examination. Sometimes the thorax and lung examinations are combined.

CHEST Exam Examples

- *No increase in AP diameter on examination.*
- *Breasts were quite nodular bilaterally, no dominant masses.*
- *Breast exam was normal.*
- *Clear to auscultation bilaterally. No rales, rubs, or crackles were noted with 3 cm distention of the diaphragm on inspiration.*
- *Breast exam deferred. Axillae revealed no palpable lymph nodes.*

Cardiovascular, Abdomen, and GU

Cardiovascular/Heart

The heart is auscultated in order to listen for the rhythm, rubs, gallops, heaves, or murmurs. The circulatory system affects all of the body's other systems, so if the heart has an abnormality, it may manifest itself in the eye exam, the neck exam, and so on. Since the examiner usually has the patient seated and has just performed the lung and/or chest exam, often the cardiac portion of the physical examination is next.

CARDIOVASCULAR Exam Examples

- *S1, S2 regular rate and rhythm without murmur, gallop, or rub. PMI is not displaced.*
- *Heart rhythm was basically regular with occasional skipped beats, no murmur.*
- *Regular rate and rhythm with a 2/4 systolic murmur.*
- *Heart exam showed a regular rhythm, normal S1 and S2, no S3 or S4, pulse of 84, blood pressure of 124/56. There was no murmur. She had good pulses in all extremities.*
- *Regular rate and rhythm with a normal S1 and a normal S2, positive S4, grade 1/6 ejection murmur at the left upper sternal border, no elevated JVD or carotid bruits.*

Abdomen

The examiner will inspect, auscultate, palpate, and percuss the abdominal area during this portion of the exam. Some physicians will incorporate the groin, rectal, anus, and genitalia exams into this portion as well. Things noted during this exam are the shape, contour, bowel sounds, and palpation of the liver, kidneys, and spleen. By palpating, muscle tone and skin turgor (tension) can be assessed.

ABDOMEN Exam Examples

- *Abdomen showed a recent left abdominal surgical scar, healing well without evidence of infection. She had high-pitched bowel sounds and mild diffuse tenderness, especially in the center of the abdomen. However, the abdomen was soft without distention. Rectal exam showed guaiac negative stool.*
- *Abdomen showed extensive scarring, scaphoid appearance, no masses or organomegaly, no tenderness, and normoactive bowel sounds. Rectal exam showed no masses, guaiac negative stool, and a small, nontender prostate.*
- *Soft with active bowel sounds, no hepatosplenomegaly.*
- *Sigmoid colon is palpable and nontender. Liver span is 9 cm. A spleen tip is palpable.*
- *Obese with no masses or bruits, no tenderness, no organomegaly. The liver edge was sharp, firm, and nontender. Rectal exam: Showed poor sphincter tone, no rectal masses, and no stool to guaiac test.*

Genitourinary

The genitourinary (GU) exam is one that assesses the reproductive organs and the urinary system. A more detailed exam might be performed in the obstetrics/gynecologic setting. In the female exam, this would include the external genitalia, female glands, vagina, cervix, meatus, perineum, and anus. In the male exam, this would include the prostate, testes, and penis.

GU Exam Examples

- *Normal circumcised male phallus with bilaterally descended testes, Foley catheter in place. Digital rectal exam deferred secondary to probable prostatitis.*
- *No history of bladder stones or kidney infections. She has tenderness over the right flank upon palpation.*
- *No penile lesions are detected.*
- *A small uterus is noted with a uterine filling defect. Vaginal discharge detected.*
- *Reducible hernia found on palpation. Descended testicles, no sign of epididymitis.*

I. **MULTIPLE CHOICE.**
   Choose the best answer.

1. Which of the following terms would be indicated under the Abdomen subheading? (◯ systolic, ◯fluid wave)

2. Which of the following terms would be indicated under the Cardiovascular/Heart subheading? (◯hepatomegaly, ◯heaves)

3. Which of the following terms would be indicated under the genitourinary subheading? (◯ perineal, ◯scaphoid)

4. Sometimes the groin, rectal, anus, and genitalia exams are including under this subheading. (◯Cardiovascular/Heart, ◯Abdomen)

5. Regurgitation is a term you would most likely hear under this subheading (◯ Cardiovascular/Heart, ◯Abdomen)

Musculoskeletal

Musculoskeletal or Extremities

The Physical Examination Musculoskeletal portion is an assessment of the muscles, bones, and joints of the body. Sometimes, the examiner will incorporate the back and/or extremities as part of this examination. A review of the movement is performed as well as inspection of hands, feet, and skin.

If not assessed and examined in the musculoskeletal section, some examiners will choose to identify the extremities on their own in the physical examination. This subheading is aptly titled EXTREMITIES.

Highlights

Some terms you might hear in the Musculoskeletal and/or Extremities section are: *range of motion, femoral pulse, popliteal pulse, pitting edema, plantar, volar, cyanosis, clubbing, edema, dorsalis pedis, lordosis, kyphosis, lumbosacral, acromegaly, rotator cuff, prosthesis, pes planus, amputation, BKA (below-knee amputation), atrophy, antalgic gait, drawer sign, torticollis, peripheral pulses, varicosities.*

MUSCULOSKELETAL/EXTREMITIES Exam Examples

- *Left knee: There is a well-healed midline scar, active range of motion 0 to 90 degrees, a mild amount of effusion, crepitus with patellar grind. The MCL (medial collateral ligament) and LCL (lateral collateral ligament) are intact with varus and valgus stressing, negative tibial sag, negative Lachman's.*
- *There is an area of edema over the posterior talofibular ligament with mild crepitus.*
- *Right knee: Well healed surgical scar, 5 degrees to 90 degrees active range of motion. Left knee: Active range of motion 0 to 130 degrees, 2+ pseudolaxity medially, negative effusion, positive patellar grind, varus malalignment, Lachman, negative pivot, tender medial joint line. Knee score, 60 degrees. Functional score, 50 degrees.*

- *Range of motion of all extremities is within normal limits.*
- *Normal examination. Pulses are 2+/4+ in the dorsalis pedis and posterior tibial.*
- *Palpation of the back reveals normal paraspinous muscle group with slight tenderness over C4.*
- *Range of motion in the hips is limited. There is a 2+ dorsalis pedis pulse on the left, and remaining peripheral pulses are absent.*
- *Range of motion is within normal limits. No evidence of venous disease or arterial disease is found.*
- *Extremities showed good pulses and perfusion. Ortolani and Barlow maneuvers were intact.*
- *The patient had +5/5 muscle strength in all 4 quadrants, +2/4 Achilles tendon reflex, +2/4 patellar reflex, and amputated toes bilaterally.*

I. MULTIPLE CHOICE.
Choose the best answer.

1. BKA stands for _____.
   - ○ below-kidney artery
   - ○ below-knee amputation
   - ○ bulbous kyphosis atrophy
   - ○ below-knee artery

2. The musculoskeletal portion of the Physical Examination is an assessment of _____.
   - ○ only the muscles of the body
   - ○ only the bones of the body
   - ○ only the joints of the body
   - ○ muscles, bones, and joints of the body

3. Which of the following is an example of something you might find under a Musculoskeletal heading?
   - ○ Palpation of the back reveals normal paraspinous muscle group with slight tenderness over C4.
   - ○ Regular rate and rhythm with a 2/4 systolic murmur.
   - ○ Carotid pulsations are equal and slight bruit is present.
   - ○ Clear to auscultation bilaterally. No rales, rubs, crackles were noted with 3 cm distention of the diaphragm on inspiration.

Neurologic and Psychiatric

Neurologic

As part of the Neurological portion of the Physical Exam, tested items will include reflexes; cranial nerves (2–12); orientation to time, place, and person (spheres); patient gait and station, and a series of signs (for example, Babinski, Romberg, Hoffman). The patient must cooperate for a majority of these tests, as this is an examination and assessment of both the central and peripheral nervous systems.

NEUROLOGIC Exam Examples

- *Cranial nerves 2–12 appeared intact. There are no deficits noted.*
- *Coordination unable to be tested. Left-sided tremor is noted consistent with previous diagnosis of Parkinson disease.*
- *Cranial nerves: The patient had no gross field cuts, but had difficulty cooperating with his fundus examination. Extraocular muscles intact. Pupils equal, round, reactive to light. Masseter is strong bilaterally. No facial asymmetry. Hearing intact grossly. Palate symmetrical bilaterally. Sternocleidomastoid and trapezoid normal. Tongue midline. Motor: 5/5 strength in all extremities proximally and distally. Tone normal times 4 extremities. No abnormal movements nor atrophy. Sensory: Intact to light touch and pinprick. Deep tendon reflexes: 2+ bilateral upper extremities, biceps, triceps, brachioradialis, 3+ knee jerks bilaterally, 1+ ankle jerks bilaterally, toes equivocal. Gait: Normal. Motor coordination and heel-to-shin grossly intact.*
- *Cranial nerves 2–12 grossly intact. Deep tendon reflexes of the biceps, triceps, and brachioradialis 2/4 bilaterally, patellar and Achilles 1+/4 bilaterally. Sensation intact in all extremities. Some hyperesthesias over left palmar surface of hand. Cerebellar, finger-to-nose good with left greater than right. Gait normal. The patient exhibits good balance. Negative Romberg.*
- *Cranial nerves 2–12 are grossly intact. His strength is 5/5 throughout. His deep tendon reflexes are symmetrical with his plantar extension reflex downgoing. There is no clonus. Pinprick and light touch are both normal. His cerebellar function is intact, showing positive finger-to-nose, heel-to-shin, rapid alternating movements are all intact. He does not have a Romberg sign. He has a slightly unsteady tandem gait and a good heel-to-toe walk.*
- *Cranial nerves 2–12 are intact. Cranial 1 not tested. Cerebellar function within normal limits. Plantar reflexes are down. Deep tendon reflexes at the knee are 2+/4 and at Achilles are 2+/4.*

Psychiatric

Often called the *Mental Status Examination*, this portion of the PE (Physical Exam) is sometimes combined with the neurological exam or is dictated separately. This portion assesses a patient's cognitive (knowledge) ability, appearance, mood, speech, and patterns of thought. Noted will be the patient's level of cooperation and attitude along with the ability or lack thereof, whether by choice or not, to answer questions. Often, this section is more detailed when dictated by an examiner affiliated with the psychiatric department of the facility.

One of the sections you can expect to encounter quite often in a psychiatric assessment is that of the DSM-IV, which is the Diagnostic and Statistical Manual of Mental Disorders. Simply stated, this breaks down the patient's assessment by axes as follows:

Axis I: Clinical disorders and syndromes
Axis II: Personality disorders (including mental retardation)
Axis III: Medical conditions (which can impact mood and emotions)
Axis IV: Psychosocial stressors (death, divorce, job loss, etc.)
Axis V: Global assessment of functioning

PSYCHIATRIC/MENTAL STATUS Exam Examples

- *The patient is a cooperative, pleasant, 53-year-old female who appears in no acute distress. Speech is rapid and mood is described as "sad." Affect is flat. She denies suicidal or homicidal ideations at the present time. She is able to perform serial 7's without difficulty. Able to name three Presidents.*

- *The patient appears older than his stated age of 43. Speech is incoherent, and the examiner was unable to assess the mental status completely due to inability of patient to cooperate.*

- *Mental Status Examination: See admission notes and discharge diagnoses are given below.*
    - *Axis I: Schizoaffective disorder, bipolar type.*
    - *Axis II: None.*
    - *Axis III: Diabetes mellitus, congestive heart failure, rheumatoid arthritis.*
    - *Axis IV: None.*
    - *Axis V: Global Assessment of Functioning (GAF) on discharge is 45.*

- *The patient is hostile and insisting he wants to go home. He states he has been "drinking a pint a day" for 48 years. He is quite adamant about wanting to leave. Four-point restraints were used and the patient refused to talk further.*

I. **FILL IN THE BLANK.**
   Using the word/word parts in the box, fill in the blanks.

   1. A term you might hear in the neurological section is

      _____.

   2. A term you might hear in the psychiatric section is

      _____.

   3. "Cranial nerves 2-12 are grossly intact" is an example of the

      _____ portion of the Physical Exam.

   4. "Speech is rapid and mood is described as sad" is an example of

      the _____ portion of the Physical Exam.

tangential
psychiatric
nystagmus
neurologic

Review: Physical Examination Subheadings

I. **SPELLING.**
   Determine if the following words are spelled correctly. If the spelling is correct, leave the word as it has already been entered. If the spelling is incorrect, provide the correct spelling.

   1. trachia midline _____
   2. nontender _____
   3. gauiac _____
   4. clonis _____
   5. carotid bruitts _____
   6. asymetric _____
   7. Romberg _____
   8. posterior tibial _____
   9. plantar _____
   10. homocidal ideation _____

II. **MULTIPLE CHOICE.**
   Choose the best answer.

   1. The subheading that covers generalities of the patient's current state is (◯Vital Signs,◯ General).

   2. The thyroid gland is assessed in the (◯Chest, ◯Neck) exam.

   3. The Vitals Signs subheadings does not typically report the patient's (◯age,◯temperature).

   4. Range of motion is typically assessed in the (◯Musculoskeletal, ◯Chest) exam.

   5. EOMs refer to the (◯eyes, ◯extremities).

6. Murmurs, rubs, and gallops are recorded in the (◯Lung, ◯Cardiovascular) exam.

7. JVD is assessed in the (◯Neck, ◯Cardiovascular) exam.

8. PERRLA is found on the (◯HEENT, ◯Abdominal) exam.

9. Lungs are usually clear to auscultation and (◯palpation, ◯percussion).

10. The term meaning no elevated temperature is (◯febrile, ◯afebrile).

Unit 5
Laboratory Data

Laboratory Data – Introduction

The laboratory data component of a medical report contains the results of lab tests that have been performed on a patient, usually to aid in confirming diagnoses, determining underlying health issues, and monitoring for such conditions as anemia, hypercholesterolemia, hyperglycemia, and electrolyte imbalances. There are many instances where lab studies are the only method to determine the etiology of patient symptoms. For instance, a patient may have feelings of lethargy and confusion with no other obvious physical symptoms. In this case, a CBC may reveal a low hemoglobin, and further iron studies may indicate that the patient is anemic. A physician might suspect anemia but could not confirm this diagnosis without the benefit of being able to perform these lab studies.

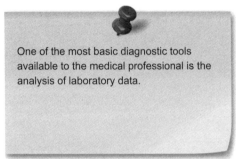

One of the most basic diagnostic tools available to the medical professional is the analysis of laboratory data.

Laboratory tests are often performed upon admission to the hospital or during checkup and followup visits to a physician's office. These laboratory values are extremely important because they provide information that can help establish or rule out diagnoses, such as anemia, diabetes, and kidney failure. Laboratory tests also allow the physician to monitor blood levels for certain medications, such as Coumadin and digoxin levels, which helps in adjusting medications to ensure the wellbeing of the patient. And finally, lab tests called toxicology screens are performed to determine the presence of drugs or poisons both in living patients and in postmortem examinations.

It is important for the working medical transcriptionist to thoroughly understand laboratory data and normal values because the results of laboratory studies are frequently cited in medical reports. The amount of laboratory data will vary from one report to another, depending upon the number and severity of a patient's medical problems. Sometimes a physician will dictate all laboratory values for any studies done; other times he/she will only dictate the abnormal values.

You are exposed to laboratory studies in several modules throughout this training program, and by the time you finish the entire training program you will have had very extensive exposure and education on laboratory data as it appears in the context of medical reports. The purpose of this unit is to provide detailed instruction on laboratory data, including laboratory abbreviations, basic laboratory studies, laboratory data in reports, and normal laboratory values.

Laboratory tests are vital to patient care, and correctly transcribed laboratory test results are equally as important. Fortunately there are a plethora of laboratory references out there (online and hard copy) to help you verify the laboratory data in medical reports!

Understanding Laboratory Data

The laboratory data portion of a medical report is a presentation of the results of diagnostic tests performed on the patient. Laboratory tests analyze the components of substances such as:

- blood
- serum
- urine
- stool
- sputum
- cerebrospinal fluid
- various other fluids
- expired air

Many medical dictionaries, such as Dorland's and Stedman's, include helpful appendices including not only the lab tests themselves, but also the normal ranges for lab values. BenchMark KB also comes with AHDI's "Normal Lab Values" Resource, an extensive database of over 250 normal lab values. That's a big help!

Most medical text documents refer to these laboratory results often by their abbreviated, usually acronymic, forms, as you will observe in the samples throughout this unit and the training program.

Again, the lab data material covered in this unit is meant to be a comprehensive overview of the laboratory data you will be exposed to as a medical transcriptionist. Diagnostic studies, in general, often include the results of x-rays, electrocardiograms, and other such procedures, as well as chemistry study results. Only the chemistry studies will be considered in this unit.

Without further ado, let's have a look at common laboratory abbreviations.

Laboratory Abbreviations

Many laboratory tests are referred to almost exclusively by their abbreviations. You will generally be required to expand abbreviations in many reports. However, even accounts that require expansion of abbreviations as a default do not necessarily require expanding the standard laboratory abbreviations. It is important, of course, that abbreviations be typed with the correct letters. You should learn what the abbreviations themselves are (ABG and not AGG, for example). It is also helpful to know what the abbreviations mean, as this understanding helps in distinguishing the letters as they are spoken.

In a medical report, you will typically find the laboratory data information in a paragraph following the Physical Examination section, although sometimes this information is given as part of the actual Physical Exam itself. Depending on the tests ordered by the treating physician(s), the results will appear in the section under the Laboratory Data heading. Of course, just as the tests ordered vary, so too will the results. In order for you to have a better understanding of laboratory data, the material contained in the following lessons will give you a better understanding of laboratory abbreviations.

By learning these abbreviations now, you will have a better understanding of what the lab tests mean, and eventually you will be able to recognize values which are normal and abnormal. It is called scaffolding—building new knowledge on top of knowledge you already have.

Laboratory Abbreviations – Lesson 1

I. **ENTER ABBREVIATIONS.**
   Enter the abbreviation and what it stands for.

   ABG: arterial blood gas
   ABGs showed a pH of 7.32, a pCO2 of 24, and a saturation of 93%.

   1. _____ (Abbreviation)

   2. _____

AFB: acid-fast bacillus
The tuberculosis pathogen is an AFB.

    3. _____ (Abbreviation)

    4. _____

BUN: blood urea nitrogen
BUN 12, creatinine 1.6.

    5. _____ (Abbreviation)

    6. _____

CBC: complete blood count
CBC revealed a WBC of 11.6, platelets of 160,000.

    7. _____ (Abbreviation)

    8. _____

CO_2: carbon dioxide
Sodium 23, CO_2 29, potassium 3.8.

    9. _____ (Abbreviation)

   10. _____

C&S*: culture and sensitivity
C&S was no growth.

   11. _____ (Abbreviation)

   12. _____

Note similarity to CNS. Both sound the same when pronounced aloud.

II. FILL IN THE BLANK.
Using the word/word parts in the box, fill in the blanks.

1. Carbon _____ was 13.

2. Creatinine was 1.2 and blood _____ nitrogen was 11.8.

3. A complete blood _____ was drawn and was within normal limits.

4. _____ blood gas revealed a pH of 7.33.

5. Culture and _____ was done.

6. Acid-fast _____ was negative.

arterial
bacillus
count
dioxide
sensitivity
urea

III. **MULTIPLE CHOICE.**
   Choose the correct term for the abbreviation expansion.

   1. CO2 – (◯common, ◯carbon) dioxide

   2. C&S – (◯culture, ◯coulture) and sensitivity

   3. ABG – (◯arterial, ◯artery) blood gas

   4. CBC – complete blood (◯culture, ◯count)

   5. BUN – blood (◯urine, ◯urea) nitrogen

Laboratory Abbreviations – Lesson 2

I. **ENTER ABBREVIATIONS.**
   Enter the abbreviation and what it stands for.

   CSF: cerebrospinal fluid
   CSF was drawn and was within normal limits.
   1. _____ (Abbreviation)
   2. _____

   FEV: forced expiratory volume
   The FEV was checked with spirometry.
   3. _____ (Abbreviation)
   4. _____

   FVC: forced vital capacity
   The FVC was also checked with spirometry.
   5. _____ (Abbreviation)
   6. _____

   H&H: hemoglobin and hematocrit
   CBC showed an H&H of 12.7 and 38.4.
   7. _____ (Abbreviation)
   8. _____

   HIV: human immunodeficiency virus
   Labs revealed HIV negative.
   9. _____ (Abbreviation)
   10. _____

KCl: potassium chloride
Kay Ciel is a trademark for a preparation of KCl.

11. _____ (Abbreviation)

12. _____

LFT: liver function test
His LFTs were grossly abnormal.

13. _____ (Abbreviation)

14. _____

II. FILL IN THE BLANK.
Enter the correct word in the blank provided.

1. His liver _____ tests were within normal limits.

2. CBC showed a _____ and hematocrit of 12.7 and 37.9.

3. She is human _____ virus negative.

4. Her _____ fluid was drawn and was within normal limits.

cerebrospinal
function
hemoglobin
immunodeficiency

III. MULTIPLE CHOICE.
Choose the correct term for the abbreviation expansion.

1. H&H – (◯humaglobin, ◯hemoglobin) and hematocrit

2. CSF – (◯cerebrospinal, ◯cerebral) fluid

3. HIV – human (◯immunodeficiency, ◯immunological) virus

4. LFT – (◯living, ◯liver) function test

Laboratory Abbreviations – Lesson 3

I. ENTER ABBREVIATIONS.
Enter the abbreviation and what it stands for.

LP: lumbar puncture
An LP was drawn and was noncontributory.

1. _____ (Abbreviation)

2. _____

O&P: ova and parasites
Stool sample was taken for O&P.

   3. _____ (Abbreviation)

   4. _____

PFT: pulmonary function test
After nebulizers, PFTs were taken.

   5. _____ (Abbreviation)

   6. _____

PSA: prostate-specific antigen
All his diagnostic data, including the PSA, indicated no recurrent disease.

   7. _____ (Abbreviation)

   8. _____

PT: prothrombin time
PT and PTT were normal.

   9. _____ (Abbreviation)

   10. _____

PTT: partial thromboplastin time
PT and PTT were normal.

   11. _____ (Abbreviation)

   12. _____

II. **FILL IN THE BLANK.**
   Enter the correct word in the blank provided.

   1. Her _____ time was normal.

   2. She had an abnormal partial _____ time.

   3. _____ puncture was normal.

   4. _____ and parasites were negative.

   5. Her pulmonary_____ tests were normal.

   6. Prostate-specific_____ is a test for prostate
      cancer.

| antigen |
| function |
| lumbar |
| ova |
| prothrombin |
| thromboplastin |

III. **MULTIPLE CHOICE.**
   Choose the correct term for the abbreviation expansion.

   1. O&P – (◯ovary, ◯ova) and parasites

   2. PFT – pulmonary (◯failure, ◯function) test

   3. PTT – (◯pulmonary, ◯partial) thromboplastin time

   4. PT – prothrombin (◯test, ◯time)

   5. PSA – prostate-specific (◯antigen, ◯antibody)

Laboratory Abbreviations – Lesson 4

   I. **ENTER ABBREVIATIONS.**
   Enter the abbreviation and what it stands for.

   RBC/rbc: red blood count/red blood cell
   UA was negative for RBCs.

   1. _____ (Abbreviation)

   2. _____

   RPR: rapid plasma reagin
   RPR was nonreactive.

   3. _____ (Abbreviation)

   4. _____

   SMA: panel of laboratory tests
   His SMA 7 was within normal limits.

   5. _____ (Abbreviation)

   6. _____

   TB: tuberculosis
   She had a positive TB test in 1973.

   7. _____ (Abbreviation)

   8. _____

   UA: urinalysis
   She had a negative UA.

   9. _____ (Abbreviation)

   10. _____

WBC/wbc: white blood count/white blood cell
CBC showed WBC 14,000, RBC 5.

11. _____ (Abbreviation)

12. _____

II. FILL IN THE BLANK.
Enter the correct word in the blank provided.

1. Her urinalysis showed no white_____ cells.

2. She had a positive_____ test in the past.

3. She had no evidence of red blood_____ in the urine.

4. She had a negative clean catch_____ .

blood
cells
tuberculosis
urinalysis

III. MULTIPLE CHOICE.
Choose the correct term for the abbreviation expansion.

1. UA – (◯urinalysis, ◯uric acid)

2. RBC – (◯real, ◯red) blood count

3. WBC – (◯white, ◯wasted) blood count

4. TB – (◯total body, ◯tuberculosis)

Basic Laboratory Studies – Lesson 1

With the laboratory abbreviations under your belt, it is time to take a look at basic lab studies. This overview of lab studies will help you put the lab abbreviations into context. Although it is not meant to be a comprehensive study of **all** laboratory tests performed, approximately 90% of the laboratory studies you will encounter as a working MT are covered here.

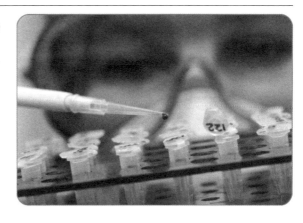

Arterial Blood Gas Study/ABG

ABGs are performed in order to test oxygen function in the lungs and how well carbon dioxide is expelled from the bloodstream. Blood is drawn from an artery and values include: pH (test for acid/alkaline base), PaO2 (oxygenation pressure measurement), PaCO2 (carbon dioxide dissolution assessment), HCO3 (bicarbonate), and SaO2 (oxygen saturation levels).

- The arterial blood gas studies are used to determine pulmonary function in patients with asthma, pneumonia, acute respiratory distress syndrome, and other respiratory ailments.
- Often included in the review of ABGs is the oxygen saturation in the blood (determined by pulse oximetry). This is presented as a percentage, with preferred values being in the mid to high 90s.

Basic Metabolic Panel/BMP

The BMP includes values for the following: Sodium, potassium, chloride, CO2, BUN (blood urea nitrogen), creatinine, glucose, calcium.

- A physician may order a BMP in order to monitor such things as electrolyte balances, kidney status, blood sugar, and calcium levels. Significant changes in these values can indicate acute problems, such as kidney failure, diabetic problems, respiratory distress, heart rhythm changes, or seizure.
- The BMP may be referred to as Chem-7 or SMA-7, although technically they are different. The BMP contains the Chem-7 values, but it also contains electrolyte values. SMA is an abbreviation derived from the equipment that processes lab samples (simultaneous multichannel autoanalyzer).

Beta HCG (human chorionic gonadotropin)

Test to determine the level of pregnancy hormones (pregnancy tests).

Cardiac Studies

CK (creatine kinase), CPK (creatine phosphokinase), CPK-MB (myocardial band enzymes of CPK), troponins.

Cardiac studies are used to determine the presence of cardiac biomarkers (enzymes, hormones, or proteins) that would indicate heart damage from events such as myocardial infarctions or coronary thromboses.

Cerebrospinal Fluid/CSF

Protein, glucose, cells.

Analysis of CSF may provide information leading to diagnosis of such conditions as trauma, meningitis, and polyneuritis. CSF is obtained by means of a lumbar puncture (LP), and the lab report may specify LP rather than CSF.

Coagulation Studies

PT/INR (prothrombin time/international normalized ratio) and PTT (partial thromboplastin time).

Coagulation studies determine the time it takes for blood to clot, and abnormal values could indicate risks for excessive bleeding or stroke. Other less common coagulation studies are done, as well.

Complete Blood Count/CBC

Leukocytes (white blood cells), hemoglobin, hematocrit, platelets, red blood cells (rbc's), MCV (mean corpuscular volume) and MCH (mean corpuscular hemoglobin), MCHC (mean corpuscular hemoglobin concentration), erythrocyte sedimentation rate (most often dictated as "sed rate").

Several types of leukocytes are identified: Myelocytes, band neutrophils (bands), segmented neutrophils (segs), lymphocytes, monocytes, eosinophils, basophils, granulocytes. The ratio of these wbc's to one another—as percentages—is called "the differential" on a CBC; the components of the differential should always add up to 100%, (although all the components may not always be dictated).

RBC can refer to either red blood count or red blood cell; WBC can refer to either white blood count or white blood cell. In lower case (rbc/wbc), the reference is nearly always to cell, not count.

The CBC measures different blood components that may indicate underlying health issues. For instance, the hemoglobin value tells how much oxygen is inside your blood cells, hematocrit details the volume of space your blood is occupying, and platelet counts determine the clotting ability of your blood. A high white blood cell count could indicate infection.

Comprehensive Metabolic Panel/CMP

Electrolytes, glucose, BUN, creatinine, albumin, total bilirubin, calcium, alkaline phosphatase (ALP), total protein (TP), AST (serum aspartate aminotransferase), ALT (alanine aminotransferase).

Notice that the comprehensive panel includes electrolytes, kidney function studies, and liver function studies, as well as glucose (blood sugar).

I. **MULTIPLE CHOICE.**
Choose the best answer.

1. A CBC is a test to determine levels of _____.
   - ○ electrolytes and creantinine
   - ○ protein and glucose
   - ○ human chorionic gonadotropin
   - ○ hemoglobin and platelets

2. If you wanted to determine if you were pregnant, you would take this test.
   - ○ Beta HCG
   - ○ BMP
   - ○ CSF
   - ○ CMP

3. This type of test includes values for pH, FEV, FVC, O2 and CO2.
   - ○ BMP
   - ○ ABG
   - ○ Cardiac Studies
   - ○ Coagulation Studies

4. This tests for CK, CPK, CPK-MB, and troponins.
   - ○ BMP
   - ○ ABG
   - ○ Cardiac Studies
   - ○ Coagulation Studies

5. Coagulation studies determine _____.
   - ○ the time it takes for blood to clot
   - ○ the amount of oxygen inside your blood cells
   - ○ a diagnosis of trauma, meningitis, and polyneritis
   - ○ blood sugar levels

6. If you wanted to find levels of bilirubin, calcium, and creatinine, you would use this test.
   ○ BMP
   ○ CMP
   ○ CBC
   ○ CSF

7. CSF is obtained by means of _____.
   ○ LP (lumbar puncture)
   ○ a blood test
   ○ urinalysis
   ○ testing saliva

8. A BMP includes values for what?
   ○ hemoglobin, hematocrit, platelets, and red blood cells
   ○ sodium, potassium, BUN, glucose, and calcium
   ○ electrolytes, BUN, calcium, total protein, and albumin
   ○ pH, FEV, FVC, O2, CO2

Basic Laboratory Studies – Lesson 2

Chem-7

Glucose, BUN, creatinine, albumin, total bilirubin, calcium, and alkaline phosphatase.

Note that the Chem-7 does not include the electrolytes.

Electrolytes (often referred to as "LYTES")

Sodium (Na), potassium (K), chloride (Cl), and bicarbonate or bicarb (CO2), magnesium (Mg or mag), and phosphates.

Electrolytes out of balance can indicate volume depletion (dehydration), over hydration, drug reactions or effects, and can be associated with certain diseases such as diabetes insipidus.

Endocrine (Diabetic)

Glucose in blood, urine. Ketones. Hemoglobin A1c (glycosylated hemoglobin).

Lab studies to determine the presence or control of diabetes mellitus.

Iron Studies

TIBC (total iron-binding capacity), serum iron, ferritin, transferrin.

Hemoglobin and hematocrit also reflect the proper balance of iron in the system. Excess iron (hemochromatosis) and deficient iron (anemia) can be indicative of major health problems.

Lipid Profile

Triglycerides, cholesterol, LDL (low-density lipids), HDL (high-density lipids).

The values reported in a lipid profile may indicate cardiac risk and predisposition to atherosclerotic heart disease. Abnormal lipid profile values could indicate the likelihood of future artery blockages. The LDL (low-density lipids) and the ratio of HDL to LDL are calculated from the results of the three main components of the panel as listed.

Liver (Hepatic) Function Tests

Albumin, total bilirubin, direct bilirubin, AST, ALT, alkaline phosphatase, LDH (lactic acid dehydrogenase), total protein.

Tests performed to evaluate and monitor liver damage.

Sometimes in complete metabolic panels or liver function testing, SGOT is used instead of AST, standing for serum glutamic-oxaloacetic transaminase, and SGPT is used instead of ALT. It stands for serum glutamic-pyruvic transaminase.

Prostate Specific Antigen/PSA

Test performed to indicate PSA levels to evaluate for possible prostate cancer or the recurrence of it.

A high PSA can indicate the presence of prostatic cancer.

Renal (or Kidney) Function Tests

BUN (blood urea nitrogen), creatinine, creatinine clearance.

These tests are performed to monitor kidney function and diagnose such conditions as renal insufficiency and chronic kidney disease.

Simultaneous Multichannel Autoanalyzer/SMA

The actual lab equipment that processes samples for analysis.

Sometimes panels of laboratory tests, such as the Chem-7, the basic metabolic panel, or the comprehensive metabolic panel, are referred to as SMA-7, SMA-12, SMA-18, and others, depending on the number of separate chemicals analyzed. All of these are tests for chemicals in the blood. You will notice that several of the items in this list include some of the same studies. The selection of laboratory studies for analysis is dependent, of course, on the medical needs of the patient.

Thyroid Function Tests

T3 uptake, T4, TSH (thyroid-stimulating hormone), thyroxine index.

Thyroid function tests are performed to determine how well the thyroid is working and are used to help diagnose hyperthyroidism (overactive thyroid) and hypothyroidism (underactive thyroid).

Urinalysis

Albumin, pH, specific gravity, rbc's, wbc's, ketones, glucose, protein, nitrites, leukocyte esterase.

Study of the chemistries in the urine can detect the presence of infection, chronic disease, dehydration, over hydration, and a variety of other illnesses and abnormalities.

I. MULTIPLE CHOICE.
Choose the best answer.

1. The test to determine the presence or control of diabetes mellitus is _____.
   - ○ Endocrine
   - ○ Lipid profile
   - ○ SMA
   - ○ Urinalysis

2. This test can indicate the presence of prostatic cancer.
   - ○ Hepatic function tests
   - ○ PSA
   - ○ SMA
   - ○ Urinalysis

3. This is the actual lab equipment that processes samples for analysis.
   - ○ SMA
   - ○ PSA
   - ○ Chem-7
   - ○ Lipid profile

4. Chem-7 does not include _____.
   - ○ creatinine
   - ○ electrolytes
   - ○ calcium
   - ○ albumin

5. This test can indicate cardiac risk and predisposition to atherosclerotic heart disease.
   - ○ Renal function tests
   - ○ PSA
   - ○ Lipid profile
   - ○ Chem-7

6. Creatinine and creatinine clearance are measured in what type of tests?
   - ○ Liver function tests
   - ○ Arterial blood gas tests
   - ○ Renal function tests
   - ○ Lipid profiles

7. Which of the following do thyroid function tests NOT test for?
   - ○ T3 uptake
   - ○ TSH
   - ○ thyroxine index
   - ○ BUN

8. Iron studies determine levels of _____.
   - ○ BUN, creatinine, creatinine clearance
   - ○ TIBC, ferritin, and transferrin
   - ○ T3 uptake, T4, thyroxine index
   - ○ triglycerides, LDL, HDL

9. Albumin, pH, specific gravity, and protein are tested for in _____.
   - ○ Chem-7
   - ○ LYTES
   - ○ Urinalysis
   - ○ Renal function

10. An electrolytes test is often referred to as _____.
    - ○ ELECTRO
    - ○ EL
    - ○ TROLYTES
    - ○ LYTES

11. Another name for liver function tests is _____.
    - ○ Thyroid function tests
    - ○ Renal function tests
    - ○ Lipid profile
    - ○ Hepatic function tests

Culture and Sensitivity

Laboratory studies, such as culture and sensitivity (C&S), detect the presence of pathogenic organisms—bacteria, viruses, yeasts, fungi, ova and parasites—as causes of disease so that effective diagnoses and treatments can be assessed and implemented.

These pathogenic organisms are **not** so easy to identify in the transcription process, mostly because they can be very challenging to spell. Note, for example, the following bacteria:

Highlights

You should notice immediately that the first element of the organism's name is capped and the second is not. The capped element of the name is the genus; the lower case element of the name is the species. If the only name given is the genus, the term is not capitalized, for example, pseudomonas or clostridium. If the genus is given as short form, such as *strep*, it should not be capitalized either.

- Stenotrophomonas maltophilia
- Escherichia coli
- Staphylococcus aureus
- Yersinia enterocolitica
- Klebsiella pneumoniae
- Actinobacillus actinomycetemcomitans

These are just a sample. There are hundreds of pathogenic organisms. (Hopefully the dictators pronounce them clearly!)

For those who want to know something more about any of these lab studies or other lab studies that we may not have included here, you can find abundant resource sites on the Internet. Here are a few to start with. These sites are good places to find the less commonly seen laboratory tests—the Cortrosyn stim (stimulation) test, immunoglobulins, D-zylose test, or antibody/antigen tests, for example.

www.labtestsonline.org

www.medicinenet.com

Review: Laboratory Studies

I. MULTIPLE CHOICE.
Choose the best answer.

1. A value not included in a CBC.
   - ◯ hemoglobin
   - ◯ hematocrit
   - ◯ sodium
   - ◯ platelets

2. Iron studies include values for serum iron, ferritin, transferrin, and ___.
   - ◯ TSH
   - ◯ TIBC
   - ◯ LDL
   - ◯ HDL

3. Test that measures blood components.

   ○ Thyroid function test
   ○ CMP
   ○ Chem-7
   ○ CBC

4. PTT is a part of a ___ study.

   ○ lipid
   ○ coagulation
   ○ glucose
   ○ urinalysis

5. Toxicology screens are performed to detect the presence of ___.

   ○ viruses
   ○ bacteria
   ○ drugs
   ○ anemia

6. The term *hyperthyroidism* means that the thyroid is ___.

   ○ overactive
   ○ underactive
   ○ appropriately active
   ○ absent

7. The terms AST and ALT are respectively interchangeable with ___.

   ○ TSH/SGTP
   ○ GGT/SGPT
   ○ SGOT/SGPT
   ○ TSH/STP

8. The abbreviation *BUN* stands for ___.

   ○ blood urea nephrology
   ○ benzolated urine nephrocytes
   ○ blood urea nitrogen
   ○ best urinalysis number

II. TRUE/FALSE.
Mark the following true or false.

1. A low hemoglobin rules out anemia.

    ○ true
    ○ false

2. Abnormal lipid profile values could indicate the likelihood of future artery blockages.

    ○ true
    ○ false

3. PSA stands for prostate-separating antigen.

    ○ true
    ○ false

4. The doctor dictates, "The patient has strep." The "s" in strep should NOT be capitalized.

    ○ true
    ○ false

Laboratory Data in Reports

In the beginning, as a new transcriptionist, understanding the laboratory data in a report may seem quite daunting. The dictator is not only using unfamiliar terms and abbreviations, but is throwing in numbers, seemingly at random. In addition, since laboratory reports are often routine, dictators tend to whip through them with amazing speed. The good news is this—because they are routine, time and experience remove the difficulty.

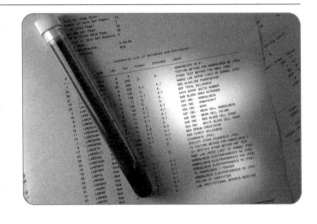

The primary objective of the following lessons is to familiarize you with the order and format of the laboratory data as it appears in medical reports. You will notice that lab reports have a style and punctuation all their own.

Complete sentences are not required. The numeric value of the test performed should be recorded either before or after the name of the test (depending on the dictation) separated by only a space. A test such as the CBC may include a variety of subtests, and you should be aware of these and how to punctuate them. As with many things in medical transcription, there is acceptable variation to how some of the laboratory information is presented. Keep that in mind as you work through this unit (and the entire training program)—it will help you keep your sanity!

The following lessons are chock full of laboratory snippets from authentic medical reports. Read through the laboratory data sections carefully and pay attention to the format and placement of the numeric values.

Lab Reports – Lesson 1

Medical Record

LABORATORY AND X-RAY FINDINGS: Her laboratory studies showed a sodium of 143, potassium of 3.8, chloride of 97, bicarbonate of 30, BUN of 9, and white count of 11,900. X-rays showed a small effusion at the left base. Abdominal films showed a normal amount of gas with no air-fluid levels.

LABORATORY DATA: White count 36.8, H&H 10.9 and 33.7. Urine showed a specific gravity of 1.031.[1] Chest x-ray showed a right upper lobe infiltrate.

LABORATORY FINDINGS: A white count was 23.7 with 41 segs and 1 band. Hemoglobin of 8.6, hematocrit of 27.3. A cath UA[2] showed 1+ blood, 30-35 white cells, and 1+ rods.

LABORATORY DATA: Initial laboratory work showed a sodium of 147, potassium 3.6, chloride 102, bicarb 32.1, glucose 136. Liver function tests were completely within normal limits. CBC showed white count of 5700,[3] H&H 11.4 and 33.6, with 287,000 platelets.

LABORATORY DATA: On admission, white blood cell count 12.8 with 5 segs, 6 bands, 83 lymphs, 5 monos, and 1 baso. Hemoglobin was 9.4, hematocrit 27.1 with platelet count of 347. VBG[4] showed pH of 7.4 and pCO2 of 34. Urinalysis was negative. Cerebrospinal fluid labs showed a protein of 61, glucose 46, no red blood cells, 4 white blood cells (1 poly, 3 lymphs). On Gram stain, there were no organisms seen. Lytes[5] were within normal limits.

Footnotes:

1. This specific gravity would be dictated as "ten thirty-one," but is transcribed correctly as 1.031.
2. A *cath* UA is one collected via catheter.
3. A number with four numerals can be transcribed with or without a comma, both 5700 and 5,700 are acceptable.
4. VBG is venous blood gas, as opposed to arterial blood gas.
5. Lytes is short for electrolytes.

I. **SPELLING.**
   Determine if the following words are spelled correctly. If the spelling is correct, leave the word as it has already been entered. If the spelling is incorrect, provide the correct spelling.

   1. sodium _____
   2. bicarbonnate _____
   3. protien _____
   4. hemoglobin _____
   5. hemotocrit _____
   6. potasium _____
   7. specific gravity _____
   8. uranalysis _____
   9. BUN _____
   10. platlets _____

Lab Reports – Lesson 2

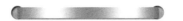

Medical Record

LABORATORY DATA: Hemoglobin 5.6, hematocrit 18, MCV 68 with MCHC of 31 and MCH 21. Liver enzymes and clotting times were normal.

LABORATORY DATA: White count 14.2 with 45 segs, 32 bands, 20 lymphs, and 3 monos. Hemoglobin was 11.2, hematocrit 34, and platelet count 286. UA was negative. Sodium was 141, potassium 4.3, chloride 98, bicarb 25, glucose 101, BUN 12, creatinine 0.3. Uric acid 3.9, phosphate 5.1, calcium 9.6, and magnesium 2.3.

LABORATORY DATA: Sodium 139, potassium 3.7, chloride 107, total CO2 of 25, creatinine 1.6, glucose 131, CPK of 257, phosphorus 2.9, alkaline phosphatase of 123, total protein 6.7, LDH 151, albumin 3.7, SGOT 23, PTT 40, PT 11.7, magnesium 2.0, total bilirubin 0.6. White cell count 7.5, hematocrit 42.1 with an MCV of 88.4, platelet count 154.

LABORATORY DATA: The urinalysis was negative. White blood cell count was 2.6, hemoglobin 11.7, MCV 93.2, platelet count 150,000. CD4 count was 35. Serum electrolytes: sodium 144, potassium 4.1, chloride 114, CO2 of 23,[1] glucose 82, creatinine 1.4, calcium 9.2, albumin 3.7, bilirubin 0.5, SGOT 62, LDH 234, SGPT 40.

LABORATORY DATA ON ADMISSION: Remarkable for a creatinine of 1.4 and a potassium of 3.5. A urinalysis shows a specific gravity of 1.015, pH 6.5, 100 protein, moderate blood, 4 white blood cells per high-powered field, and 9 red blood cells per high-powered field. Discharge labs are significant for a creatinine of 2.2 and a hematocrit of 31.6.

Footnotes:

1. Even if dictated simply as CO2 23, it is generally preferred to put "of" between the consecutive numbers 2 and 2.

I. **MULTIPLE CHOICE.**
   Choose the correct term for the abbreviation expansion.

   1. MCV – mean (◯corpuscular, ◯cortical) volume

   2. CO2 – carbon (◯dioxide, ◯dating)

   3. BUN – blood (◯urine, ◯urea) nitrogen

   4. PT – (◯prothrombin, ◯partial) time

   5. PTT – partial (◯thromboplastin, ◯thrombolitic) time

Lab Reports – Lesson 3

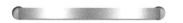

LABORATORY AND X-RAY FINDINGS: She had initially a white blood cell count of 15.7, H&H of 11.9 and 35.6. BUN and creatinine were within normal limits. Her urinalysis showed 3+ bacteria, 2+ occult blood. Urine culture grew out E. coli greater than 100,000 organisms. Followup labs showed white blood cell count climbing to 29,000, and after treatment lowered to 19,000. A followup urine culture did not grow out any E. coli after antibiotic treatment.

LABORATORY AND X-RAY FINDINGS: Chest x-ray on admission showed a large consolidation of the right upper lobe with a questionable infiltrate versus atelectasis in the right middle lobe. His white count was 16.5 with 44 segs, 44 bands, and 10 lymphocytes. His hemoglobin was 13.4, hematocrit 39.9, platelet count 227. Urine showed a specific gravity of 1.012 with 1+ blood, 1+ protein. Electrolytes were remarkable for a slightly low potassium of 3.2. His liver function studies and amylase were normal. ABGs showed pH of 7.4, pCO2 and pO2 within normal ranges.

LABORATORY AND X-RAY FINDINGS: Chest x-ray shows a left upper lobe pneumonia. Blood cultures were drawn. Glucose 125, sodium 144, potassium 5.3, chloride 97, CO2 29, BUN 11, creatinine 0.2. White blood cell count was 58.9, hemoglobin 10.2, hematocrit 33.0, differential showing 55 segs, 16 bands, 23 lymphs, and 3 monos. UA: specific gravity 1.024, 0-1 white blood cells, and 0-1 RBCs. Spinal fluid showed 2 polys, 4 RBCs. Gram stain: 3+ protein.

LABORATORY DATA: Chem-7 unremarkable. White blood count 8.7, hemoglobin 13.1, hematocrit 39.4, platelets 728,000, MCV 113, macrocytosis 2+. Calcium, magnesium, phosphorus essentially normal. LFTs normal. CSF studies showed glucose and protein within normal limits.

I. MATCHING.
Match the correct term to the definition.

1. ____ Hidden, obscure, not obvious on observation.

2. ____ Sugar.

3. ____ Sodium, potassium, chloride, bicarbonate.

4. ____ Incomplete expansion of a lung or portion of a lung.

5. ____ A chemical in the blood or urine that is used in the diagnostic analysis of kidney function.

6. ____ A condition characterized by larger than normal erythrocytes.

7. ____ Disk-shaped structures found in blood that help coagulate blood.

8. ____ Segmented neutrophils, lymphocytes, monocytes.

A. atelectasis
B. macrocytosis
C. occult
D. platelets
E. creatinine
F. glucose
G. electrolyte
H. white blood cells

Normal Laboratory Values

As a medical transcriptionist, you must have at least a general understanding of normal laboratory values. There may be times when an author dictates a value mistakenly, and, as an efficient medical transcriptionist, it is up to you to catch these types of errors and bring them to the attention of QA or the client, depending on the procedure followed by your employer. Lab value errors can adversely affect patient care, so it is of the utmost importance that the values be reported correctly. In this lesson, we will look at normal values for some of the more common tests. This list is not meant to be comprehensive by any means, but it will cover values that will frequently pop up during your career as an MT. We have also included some notes that may be helpful along the way. Normal ranges that differ from male to female are notated with M and F.

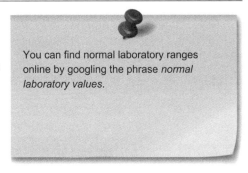

You can find normal laboratory ranges online by googling the phrase *normal laboratory values*.

Frequently Dictated CBC Components

Lab Test	Normal Range	Information
White Blood Cell Count (WBC)	3800–11,000 (may be expressed as 3.8–11.0 thousand)	High levels usually indicate bacterial infection.
Neutrophils	50%–81%	High levels may indicate active infection.
Lymphocytes	14%–44%	Elevated level may indicate viral infection.
Monocytes	2%–6%	Elevated level may indicate chronic infection or cancer.

Eosinophils	1%–5%	Elevated level may indicate allergic reaction or parasites.
Basophils	0%–1%	Elevated level may indicate allergic reaction or chronic inflammation.
Red blood cells (rbc's)	M 4.2–5.6, F 3.8–5.1	If rbc's are low, then hemoglobin and hematocrit (H&H) will most likely also be low.
Hemoglobin	M 14–18 g/dL, F 12–16 g/dL	Amount of O2 carrying protein in blood, gives blood red color. Low level indicates anemia.
Hematocrit	M 39%–54%, F 34%–47%	Percentage of blood that is occupied by red blood cells. Low level may indicate anemia.
Platelets	140,000–450,000 /ml	Platelets play an important role in blood clotting.

Frequently Dictated CMP Components

Lab Test	Normal Range	Information
Sodium	135–148 mEq/L	Low levels (hyponatremia) may lead to seizures or other neurological problems.
Potassium	3.5–5.5 mEq/L	Elevation (hyperkalemia) can indicate renal failure or diabetes; low levels (hypokalemia) can lead to heart arrhythmia.
Chloride	96–112 mEq/L	Abnormal levels may indicate kidney problems.
CO2 (or bicarbonate)	22–30 mmol/L	Helps to maintain acidity level in bodily fluids.
BUN	6–23 mg/dL	Elevated levels may indicate such events as heart failure, excessive protein intake, or that the kidneys are just not functioning properly.
Creatinine	0.6–1.5 mg/dL	Low or high levels could indicate kidney damage.
Glucose	65–99 mg/dL	Sustained elevation above normal range may indicate diabetes. Below normal range is hypoglycemia, and above normal range is hyperglycemia.
Calcium	8–11 mg/dL	Calcium is important for such processes as proper cardiac function, bone metabolism, and protein absorption.
AST (SGOT)	< 35 IU/L (ideal 20-48)	
ALT (SGPT)	< 35 IU/L	

Frequently Dictated Lipoproteins and Triglycerides

Lab Test	Normal Range
Cholesterol, total	< 200 mg/dL
HDL cholesterol	30–70 mg/dL

| LDL cholesterol | 65–180 mg/dL |
| Triglycerides | 45–155 mg/dL (< 160) |

Review: Normal Laboratory Values

I. **MULTIPLE CHOICE.**
   Choose the best answer.

1. The physician dictates what sounds like the following: "WBC 9000, hemoglobin 46, hematocrit 39, platelets 263,000." Which value is likely incorrect (misstated or misunderstood)?
   ○ WBC
   ○ hemoglobin
   ○ hematocrit
   ○ platelets

2. The following is dictated for CMP results, but the blanked word cannot be understood in the dictation: "Sodium 139, potassium 4.2, chloride 99, CO2 29, BUN 15, ___ 0.9, glucose 98, calcium 9." Ruling out all other possibilities and listening to the dictation again, what would the most likely missing component be?
   ○ hemoglobin
   ○ iron
   ○ creatinine
   ○ alkaline phosphatase

3. Which of the following values would be considered normal?
   ○ hemoglobin 13
   ○ BUN 40
   ○ glucose 240
   ○ creatinine 2.9

4. The physician dictates, "WBC 8300, H&H 13.7 and 37.2, respectively." The hematocrit value is ___.
   ○ 13.7
   ○ 37.2
   ○ 8300
   ○ None of the above

5. A patient with a glucose of 266 would be considered ___.
   ○ anemic
   ○ cachectic
   ○ hypoglycemic
   ○ hyperglycemic

II. TRUE/FALSE.
Mark the following true or false.

1. A patient with a WBC of 3800 almost certainly has a bacterial infection.
   - ○ true
   - ○ false

2. Hyperkalemia means an elevated potassium level.
   - ○ true
   - ○ false

3. Hyponatremia may lead to seizures.
   - ○ true
   - ○ false

4. A total cholesterol level of 225 is considered to be within normal range.
   - ○ true
   - ○ false

5. An elevated creatinine could indicate kidney problems.
   - ○ true
   - ○ false

Laboratory Data Helpful Tips

The new MT may find laboratory data particularly daunting; but be assured that it gets easier with experience. Transcription of laboratory data will eventually become almost second nature. There are a few important tips to remember to help you transcribe laboratory data with accuracy and efficiency.

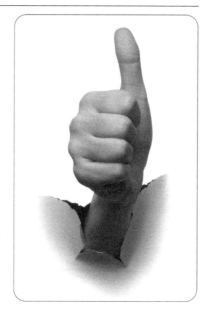

Critical Concepts for Lab Data Success

- **Never guess** at a laboratory value. Keep in mind that patients are receiving treatment based on these values, and incorrect values could adversely affect patient care, possibly leading to incorrect medication doses and even death of a patient.
- Question dictated values if they are far out of line with normal or abnormal ranges. For example, if you think the physician is dictating a creatinine of 380, be sure to question it by following the appropriate process recommended by your employer. Remember, physicians are human and they can make mistakes, too. It is always safer to question a value rather than to just transcribe incorrect information.
- You may find it helpful to keep a comprehensive printout of normal laboratory values handy, because dictated laboratory components vary from client to client, physician to physician.

Unit 6
Formatting Guidelines

Formatting – Introduction

Rules, standards, and *preferences*: These are but a few of the words you will encounter when your future employer, company, or client utilizes your services as a transcriptionist. The rules, standards, and preferences of how the document is prepared are all a part of the formatting process we will be covering in this unit.

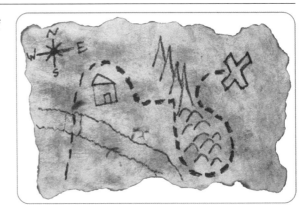

Merriam-Webster defines format as "a method of organizing data…the general plan of arrangement or choice of material." Quite simply, formatting is a facet of medical transcription that further enhances the integrity, quality, and consistency of the document with that of the proposed standard/style.

Imagine you are taking your dog for a walk and a passer-by in an SUV flags you down to ask for directions to an area theater. He has a pen and paper handy, so you take the time to explain how to get there and draw an outline reflecting his path of travel. You might use octagons for stop signs, arrows to indicate turns, and squares to indicate buildings. On the other hand, I might use circles for stop signs, dotted lines to indicate a path, and forego the use of landmarks in order to get the lost driver to his destination. The way the map is drawn and the details that went into its creation are, rough though they might be, formatting styles.

Similarly, in medical transcription Account A might insist that all reports be transcribed verbatim, meaning word for word. Account B, however, might require reports to be edited with a specific set of guidelines in place. Spelling and grammatical errors, idiomatic phrases and expressions, as well as slang phrases and lab data language are all areas that might be affected by account-specific instructions, or formatting preferences.

Medicine, like all aspects of life, evolves and changes. It is impossible to create a unit in which all-inclusive instructions are given in terms of medical document formatting. What we can do, however, is provide an overview of the types of styles, rules, and formatting specifics you might encounter when transcribing. Your future employer will provide you with specifics in order to apply these styles and preferences to the documents you transcribe.

Formatting and Industry Trends

The format of a medical report will vary according to the individual client. Your future employer will provide you with account specifications (also known as account instructions). Part of your job is to ensure these rules and specifications are carried out and adhered to properly. Although all rules are subject to change from specific clients, there are general industry guidelines that apply to all of medical transcription (unless specifically contraindicated by the client). These include things such as medications, dates, abbreviations, usage and placement of numbers, and so forth. An overview of these style issues will be provided in this unit.

There are medical transcription industry standards, practices, and trends that, fortunately for you, will never change and are quite static in their very nature. For example, it is generally unacceptable to begin a sentence with a number, as illustrated below.

> **Dictated:** 12 days ago, the patient began to feel sluggish, diaphoretic, and lightheaded.
>
> **Transcribed:** Twelve days ago, the patient began to feel sluggish, diaphoretic, and lightheaded.

Remember those exceptions you read about? Some clients might allow a sentence to begin with a year: "2007 was the doctor's busiest year so far." However, some might prefer and allow the transcriptionist to

86

recast the sentence: "The doctor's busiest year so far was 2007." Within this context, you will be instructed as to whether *flagging* is necessary in such situations. *Flagging* is an account-specified way to highlight or draw attention to a potential error, missing data, indistinguishable information, or even inconsistent information. Again, the company that employs you will have a specific protocol in place for handling such situations and how they will expect you to adhere to the protocol.

All of this may seem a bit overwhelming at this point. You might be thinking, how am I supposed to remember all of these terms, forms, standards, procedures, rules, and now exceptions to those rules? If you can read, write, and speak English (and we know you can) then you've already mastered one of the most difficult languages to learn in the world. The beauty of that is you will be applying your knowledge of English, verbs agreement, tenses, commas, etc. to medical transcription. Medicine evolves and there are aspects of it that are ever-changing. English language rules are, for the most part, set in stone. Recall the lost traveler at the beginning of this lesson and the map you drew. Like your map, client A might want their formatting done according to one set of rules while client B might want a slight variation on those rules. Having those documents handy to refer to as you learn account instructions will help you tremendously. For now, having an overview of what to expect and what those rules, standards, and specifications might look like is a good starting point.

General Formatting Rules

In general, there are some industry rules or trends that rarely change according to account or client. Bear in mind there are always exceptions, but for the most part these are general rules you will be expected to adhere to as a medical transcriptionist. (Consider these sort of the default styles for the industry.)

Abbreviations

Do not use abbreviations in any diagnosis lists (admission, discharge, pre/postoperative), impressions, or lists/names of procedures and operations. For example, if in the list of diagnoses a doctor states, "TIA," and you can be 100% certain that this means transient ischemic attack by the content/context of the report, you would instead transcribe "transient ischemic attack" in place of TIA.

Never abbreviate a word that a doctor dictates in full. Although tempting to shorten a word into an abbreviation to save keystrokes and get done quicker, do not do so. For example, if a doctor states "myocardial infarction," do **not** transcribe MI.

Abbreviations **are** to be used for metric units of measure used in medical reports when a numeric quantity precedes the unit of measure. For example, "A 2-cm lesion was located" or "Her blood pressure was 120/80 mmHg." Never add an "s" to pluralize a metric unit of measure.

Slang

Transcribe in full any slang terms. Doctors use slang terms often in medical reports. Examples are: alk phos is 78 (instead of alkaline phosphatase), an appy in 1984 (instead of appendectomy), and scope was withdrawn (instead of laryngoscope or some other kind of scope). **Unless otherwise instructed**, you are to transcribe the full and appropriate word or words. (It should be noted that we say "unless otherwise instructed" because verbatim transcription is becoming more and more common in the industry—which means more and more slang is being transcribed as dictated.)

Flags

Some words are to be flagged, omitted, or left blank. Obscenities, derogatory remarks, and double entendres (words that have varied meanings, one of which could be perceived as inappropriate or insensitive) are all examples of types of language that should be avoided. In general, obscene words are not to be used unless instructed by the client (or in many cases, part of a direct quotation).

Brief Forms

Use brief forms only when dictated. A brief form is a word that has been shortened and is acceptable as a shortened version. Some of the most common of these are exam, prepped, Pap smear, temp, and sed rate. These are acceptable only if they are dictated as such. I know what you are thinking—what makes one word slang and another a brief form? Unfortunately and fortunately, if things like slang versus brief forms are not outlined specifically by your account instructions, there will be acceptable variation to how you present this type of information.

mmHg

The abbreviation for millimeters of mercury is mmHg. This is a common term used with pressure readings, such as blood pressure and tourniquet pressure. If you do abbreviate it, you should use the correct form, which is mmHg. A period is not to be used unless mmHg falls at the end of a sentence.

Dictated: The patient's blood pressure was 113 over 84 millimeters of mercury.

Transcribed: The patient's blood pressure was 113/84 mmHg.

Dictated: Her pressure was 139 over 69 millimeters of mercury earlier and it has since normalized.

Transcribed: Her pressure was 139/69 mmHg earlier and it has since normalized.

pH

NEVER capitalize the p in pH. The term pH is used to designate alkalinity and it should **NEVER** be capitalized. If it is dictated first in a sentence, add the word "the" or recast the sentence, according to client/account instructions.

Dictated: ph was 7.3.

Transcribed: The pH was 7.3.

Dates

Dates are to be written out unless otherwise specified. Your client will probably have a preference for the way dates are designated; for example, in the military they are entered as day/month/year in the following manner: 10 Feb 93. It can also be appropriate to transcribe as 2-10-93 or 2/10/93, if so requested. But, if there is no specific requirement, dates should be spelled out in the body of a report, as in February 10, 1993. The good news—the patient information has been washed from the practicum reports in this training program in order to protect patient confidentiality. This means you will not be transcribing dates in our practicum. It is important for you to understand, however, that there are a number of ways to correctly present dates.

Allergies

If a patient has allergies, a special font or format is usually used in order to draw attention to them. Some accounts/clients prefer all caps for allergies, as in: ALLERGIES: ERYTHROMYCIN AND ASPIRIN. Others may use italics, special formatting, or any form of character encoding so that allergies are clearly distinguished and alerted from the rest of the report contents.

Numbers

When transcribing numbers the issues are whether to use Arabic versus Roman and whether to spell out the number (for example, seven) or use the numeral (7) instead. Within this unit, specifics as to the preferred usage of numbers will be examined. In general, most numbers that you will transcribe will be Arabic unless Roman is the usage mandated, and most numbers will be presented as the numerals instead of being spelled out (again, this is just in general).

I. **TRUE/FALSE.**
   Mark the following true or false.

1. All transcribed medical reports follow the same set of standards for formatting.

   ○ true
   ○ false

2. In medical transciption, it is generally not accepted to begin a sentence with a number.

   ○ true
   ○ false

3. Flagging is a way of passing a report on to another transcriptionist to finish.

   ○ true
   ○ false

4. Slang terms should always be transcribed exactly as they are dictated.

   ○ true
   ○ false

5. The abbreviation mmHg is the appropriate abbreviation for millimeters of mercury.

   ○ true
   ○ false

Book of Style

One of the references you will encounter in the industry is called the *Book of Style for Medical Transcription*, which is a stylistic and practical book of guidelines and preferences dealing with medical transcription, its informational points of grammar, punctuation, and usage. The Book of Style is a product of the Association for Healthcare Documentation Integrity (AHDI), formerly known as American Association for Medical Transcription (AAMT). As stated earlier, there are many styles and variations in formatting that will be presented to you in your training and eventual employment as a medical transcriptionist, and the Book of Style is one of them. The Book of Style is included in the KB Benchmark tool. We will refer to some of the standards within that context in this section of the formatting unit. (Of note, the information in this unit is based on the *BOS 3E*, the *Book of Style for Medical Transcription, 3rd Edition*.)

You may want to refer back to this unit after you have had an opportunity to practice and work through the medical transcription content. For now, take the time to review these standards and be aware that there are acceptable variations and your future employer(s) and accounts will provide instruction and specifics detailing their preferences.

Acronyms and Initialisms

The pages contained in this lesson will outline an array of Book of Style standards. The exercises incorporated into the lesson will test your knowledge of the material presented. All quoted material indicates AHDI BOS 3E as the reference source.

Acronyms

Acronyms are abbreviations formed from the initial letters of each of the successive words (or major parts of a compound term or selected letter of a word or phrase) that is pronounced as a single word.

Some examples of medical and non-medical acronyms:

- AIDS – acquired immune deficiency syndrome
- GERD – gastroesophageal reflux disease
- CABG – coronary artery bypass graft
- LIMA – left internal mammary artery
- OSHA – Occupational Safety and Health Administration
- SADD – Students Against Drunk Driving

Some acronyms derived from initial letters are NOT capitalized. Examples of some are:

- scuba – self-contained underwater breathing apparatus
- laser – light amplification by stimulated emission of radiation
- radar – radio detection and ranging

Acronyms are to be transcribed as dictated unless otherwise indicated or instructed.

Initialisms

An **initialism** is similar to an acronym in that it is "formed from the initial letter of each of the successive words (or major parts of a compound term or of selected letters of a word or phrase) that is **not** pronounced as a word, but by each letter." This is easy to remember because an initialism is just that, a grouping of initials that you would **not** say aloud as you would an acronym.

Some examples of medical and non-medical initialisms:

- CPR – cardiopulmonary resuscitation
- VCR – videocassette recorder
- R&D – research and development
- LMP – last menstrual period
- GFM – good fetal movement
- CBBB – complete bundle branch block
- BGRS – blood glucose reagent strip

Abbreviations and Brief Forms

Abbreviations

An **abbreviation** is a shortened form of a word or a phrase that is used in place of the whole. Abbreviations are prevalent in the world of medicine. According to BOS 3, it is generally preferred to write out an abbreviation or acronym in full if it is used in the admission, discharge, preoperative, or postoperative diagnosis; in the consultative conclusion; or in the operative title. Non-disease-entity abbreviations accompanying diagnostic and procedure statements may be used if dictated. (It is preferable to abbreviate units of measure.) When you are

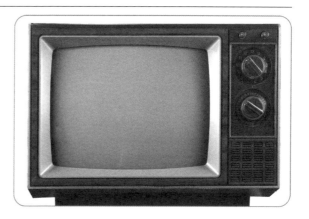

unable to translate an abbreviation or shortened form within one of these sections, you would normally flag it for attention.

Examples of abbreviations:

- WBC (white blood count)
- USMC (United States Marine Corps)
- t.v. (television)
- TB (tuberculosis)

State and territory names should be abbreviated if they are preceded by a city, a state, or a territory name. States should be abbreviated in an address. Names of states, territories, and countries should not be abbreviated if they are used alone. The following illustrate some examples of this rule:

My brother was taken to an operating room in Kansas City, MO, when we visited recently.

I am looking forward to seeing the specialist in California.

Drug Terminology Abbreviations and Punctuation

Drug dosages are often abbreviated and kept "as is," when transcribing. The following list should **not** be translated/expanded.

Abbreviation	English Translation
a.c.	before food
b.i.d.	twice a day
gtt.	drops (preferred if you spell out drops)
n.p.o.	nothing by mouth
n.r.	do not repeat
p.c.	after food
p.o.	by mouth
p.r.n.	as needed
q.4 h.	every 4 hours (note the space: q.4 h. is used for clarity)
q.h.	every hour

q.i.d.	4 times a day
t.i.d.	3 times a day
u.d.	as directed

Brief Forms

Brief forms are commonplace in medical transcription. Some are acceptable and some are not. Brief forms are simply shortened forms of words. Brief forms are to be transcribed as dictated unless they appear in headings, diagnoses, and operative titles. You should lowercase the brief form unless it is routinely capitalized. An ending period is not used, and the plural of a brief form is accomplished by adding the letter *s* without an apostrophe. On the job, some of your accounts may prefer expansion of brief forms, and some brief forms are not acceptable at all.

Examples of some brief forms both medical and non-medical:

- phone
- Pap smear
- exam
- segs
- cath
- infarct
- fax
- temp

Review: Acronyms, Initialisms, Abbreviations, and Brief Forms

I. **MULTIPLE CHOICE.**
   Choose the best answer.

1. An example of an acronym is ___.
   ○ WBC
   ○ p.r.n.
   ○ CPR
   ○ CABG

2. The abbreviation p.o. translates to ___.
   ○ by mouth
   ○ as needed
   ○ every morning
   ○ before food

3. An initialism is ___.
   ○ A shortened form of a word or a phrase which is used in place of the whole.
   ○ A grouping of initials that you would NOT say aloud as you would an acronym.
   ○ Formed from the initial letters of words or major parts of a compound term.
   ○ Sometimes known as brief forms.

4. The word *temp* in medical terminology is an example of a/an ___.
   - ○ abbreviation
   - ○ brief form
   - ○ initialism
   - ○ acronym

5. Twice a day would be transcribed as ___.
   - ○ b.i.d.
   - ○ t.i.d.
   - ○ t.a.d.
   - ○ n.p.o.

II. MATCHING.
Match the abbreviation with the appropriate translation.

1. ___ do not repeat
2. ___ as directed
3. ___ after food
4. ___ every hour
5. ___ drops

A. q.h.
B. u.d.
C. n.r.
D. gtt.
E. p.c.

Eponyms

What the dictator may say: After parturition, the patient complained of alopecia, cephalgia, and pain over the cicatrix. The on-call attending ordered lab tests of FSH in addition to testing the hypophysis.

What the dictator means: After childbirth, the patient complained of hair loss, headache, and pain over the scar. The on-call attending ordered lab tests of FSH, follicle-stimulating hormone, in addition to testing the pituitary gland.

Question: Why don't dictators just speak in plain English?

Answer: Because this isn't plain English—it's the medical language. As medical transcriptionists we have to know what the doctor means. Patient document integrity, risk management, and quality assurance, all depend on it.

An **eponym** is a name, such as drug, disease, operation, or anatomic structure, based on or derived from a person or a place. The BOS 3E prefers and recommends dropping the apostrophe s ('s). Examples of some medical eponyms are:

- Alzheimer disease
- Down syndrome
- Parkinson disease
- Cushing syndrome
- Addison disease

- Pap (Papanicolaou) smear
- Apgar score
- Hodgkin lymphoma
- Gram stain
- Arnold-Chiari malformation
- Guillain-Barre syndrome
- Crohn disease
- Klatskin tumor

Exceptions to the Eponym Rule:

HOWEVER—and that is capitalized because this is really important—not every apostrophe s ('s) is dropped in eponyms. While the possessive form remains an acceptable alternative, BOS indicates the use of an apostrophe s as preferred by client or employer. Further, some eponyms end in the letter s, and in those cases, the s is to be kept in place. Examples are:

- Homans sign
- Christmas factor
- Bundle of His
- Pouch of Douglas
- Pores of Kohn
- Brill-Symmers disease
- Libman-Sacks disease
- Riggs disease
- Williams syndrome

Unfortunately, there is no magic wand to wave and commit these instantaneously to memory. Your on-the-job experience and hands-on dictation practicum will benefit you greatly in successfully embracing the sometimes possessive nature of medicine.

Slang

Dictators frequently use **slang**, **jargon**, or **shortened forms**, and we hardly even recognize them as such because they have become so commonplace. While abbreviated forms are often acceptable, the same thing is not necessarily true of slang. In formal medical documents it is better to avoid slang terms and phrases unless the meaning cannot be determined otherwise (which is a very rare occurrence) or when they more accurately communicate the meaning (also a rare occurrence). The BOS states, in general, to avoid slang phrases except when they are essential to the report, when they more accurately communicate the meaning than their translation would, or when their meaning cannot be determined.

Slang	Expanded Form
a-fib, A-fi, AFib	atrial fibrillation
alk phos	alkaline phosphatase
appy	appendectomy or appendicitis
bicarb	bicarbonate
bili	bilirubin
CBC with diff	CBC (complete blood count) with differential
caps	capsules
cath	catheter or catheterization

chemo	chemotherapy
chole	cholecystectomy
crit	hematocrit
DC	discontinue or discharge
detox	detoxification
dig	digoxin or digitalis
dip sesta	dipyridamole sestamibi
double J stent	JJ stent
echo	echocardiogram
eos	eosinophils
flex sig	flexible sigmoidoscopy
Foley	Foley catheter
HCTZ	hydrochlorothiazide
hem/onc	hematology/oncology
hep C (A, B)	hepatitis C (A, B)
K	potassium
KCl	potassium chloride
lac	laceration
lymphs	lymphocytes
lytes	electrolytes
mag	magnesium
meds	medications
mg	milligrams
mcg	micrograms
monos	monocytes
nebs	nebulizers
neuro	neurological or neurology
neuropsych	neuropsychiatry
O2 sat	oxygen saturation
path	pathology
perf	perforation
preop	preoperative
postop	postoperative
prepped	prepared
psych	psychiatry or psychology

pulse ox	pulse oximetry
regurg	regurgitation
rehab	rehabilitation
sat	saturation
sed rate	sedimentation rate
segs	segmented neutrophils
t. bili	total bilirubin
tabs	tablets
triple A, AAA	abdominal aortic aneurysm
V-tach	ventricular tachycardia
voc rehab	vocational rehabilitation

Review: Eponyms and Slang

I. **MULTIPLE CHOICE.**
   Choose the best answer.

   1. The correct expanded form for mcg is (◯micrograms, ◯milligrams).

   2. Slang for perforation is often called (◯perfo, ◯perf).

   3. (◯Alzheimer, ◯Alzheimer's) disease affects a person's memory and cognition.

   4. KCl is an abbreviation for (◯potassium nitrate, ◯potassium chloride).

   5. CBC with diff means CBC with (◯difference, ◯differential).

   6. The (◯bundle of Hi's, ◯bundle of His) deals with the conduction system of the heart.

   7. An appendectomy or appendicitis is sometimes called (◯appy, ◯append) in slang.

   8. Dip sesta is slang for (◯dypyridamole sestamibi, ◯dipyridamole sestamibi).

   9. Pap smear is an example of a/an (◯eponym, ◯synonym).

   10. Saturation is sometimes called (◯sat, ◯sit) in slang.

Dangerous Abbreviations

The Institute for Safe Medication Practices (ISMP) has designated a list of abbreviations that are deemed dangerous to the patient's safety according to how they are transcribed. This list appears in your BOS 3E pages 206–213. You can also find a PDF copy of the ISMP Dangerous Abbreviations list by visiting the following link: www.ismp.org/newsletters/ambulatory/issues/abbreviations.pdf.

With BenchMark KB, you have access to a quality alerts library, including the Joint Commission and ISMP dangerous abbreviations and recommendations. Common transcription style and critical alerts are housed here. It's not a bad idea to check it out!

Numbers

The trend in medical transcription is to steer away from the use of Roman numerals and to use Arabic numbers instead (unless your company, client, or account specifies their usage). Arabic numerals are 0 through 9.

Some things to keep in mind when transcribing numbers according to BOS:

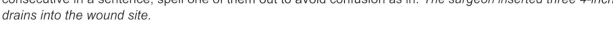

Arabic numbers are to be used as opposed to transcribing the numbers spelled out.
For example, *The patient was rushed to the emergency room within 30 minutes of the accident.*
Exception: When there are 2 numbers which are consecutive in a sentence, spell one of them out to avoid confusion as in: *The surgeon inserted three 4-inch drains into the wound site.*

When transcribing units of measurement, use the Arabic numeral and abbreviate the measurement.
For example, it should be *5 mg*, *10 mm*, *150 mg*, etc. NOT *ten mm* or *5 millimeters.*

Express a ratio with the number and a colon.
For example, *head circumference to abdominal circumference ratio is 1:2.*

Express a range with the word "to" or a hyphen.
For example, *his blood sugars ranged from 78-123* OR *78 to 123.*

Use a hyphen to express suture size.
This may also be designated by the correct number of zeros, but is more difficult to read: *0000000000 suture for eye surgery.*
A suture is defined by a certain number of zeros (designating the thickness of the suture material: the larger the number, the smaller the diameter of the suture material). For example, *We used 3-0 Vicryl to close the skin.*

Use Arabic digits to number vertebrae and intervertebral spaces.
For example, *She had an L4-5 spondylolisthesis. She had a T3 compression fracture.*
Of note, some clients will delineate vertebrae with hyphens, others with commas: *L4-5; L4,5; T10-11; T10,11.* The hyphenated form is generally preferred, however. It is preferable to repeat the vertebral letter before each vertebra listed, as in: *The herniation involves C5, C6, and C7.*

When using a slash in place of the word per, also abbreviate the units of measurement.
For example, do not type *15 milligrams/second*, but *15 mg/sec.*

Use Arabic digits with symbols, abbreviations, and laboratory values.
For example, *CO2 38, pH 7.3, LDH 7, alkaline phosphatase 73.*

Use digits with units of measurement.:
For example, *The specimen was 4 cm x 6 cm x 2 cm.*

Use a zero digit and a decimal to designate values of less than one, but do not ADD a decimal and zero for values of one or greater,.
For example, *0.25% lidocaine was used, but not 120.0 cc of fluid was given.*

Transcribe a blood pressure reading with numbers and a slash.
For example, *Blood pressure was 113/73.*

Use Arabic digits to designate Apgar scores.
For example, *Apgars were 8 and 9.* (This is the visual test performed on a newborn infant at one and five minutes)

Roman numerals are used to express stages with a few exceptions.
Periods are not to be used with Roman numerals, and they are to be capitalized unless otherwise directed. Examples of usage and exceptions:

A stage II decubitus ulcer
A stage 2 femoral neck Garden fracture
Cancer of the left ovary, FIGO stage III

Cranial nerves may be Arabic or Roman.
Cranial nerve notation is according to client specifications, as in *cranial nerves 2-12* or *cranial nerves II-XII.*

Ordinal numbers indicate position or order in a series.
Examples include *4th rib*, *8th month of pregnancy*, the *6th cranial nerve*. BOS recommends their usage be in numeric form and not spelled out.

Plurals and numbers.
An apostrophe s ('s) is used to form a plural of a single-digit number, as in *4 x 4's*. However, add an s without an apostrophe to pluralize multiple-digit numbers, as in: *30s, 1960s*.

Percentage and numbers.
Use arabic numbers before the % sign when transcribing, as in *60%*. Do not place a space between the number and the % sign.

If a number begins the sentence, write out the number and write out percent, as in *Twelve percent of the patients were randomized in the study.*

If the amount is under 1%, then place a zero before the decimal, as in *0.4%* and not *.4%*.

If a range of values is given, repeat the % or the word percent with each value, as in

The lab values decreased from 59% to 40% in the last hour.
Four percent to eight percent of the patients had the flu.

Use decimals and not fractions when using percents, as in *0.5%* and not *½%*.

Be certain the subject and verb agree according to the wording. *Percent of* takes a singular verb when the word following *of* is singular. It takes a plural verb when the word following *of* is plural, as in:

Eighty percent of the eyelid was infected.
Fifteen percent of the patients saw the doctor on Wednesday.

When percent stands alone and is not followed by the word *of*, it takes on a singular verb, as in: *Six percent is inadequate.*

Review: Dangerous Abbreviations and Numbers

I. **TRUE/FALSE.**
   Mark each of the following true or false according to Book of Style requirements.

   1. The correct way to transcribe qhs is q.h.s.
      ○ true
      ○ false

   2. An apostrophe s ('s) is used to form a plural of a single-digit number.
      ○ true
      ○ false

   3. Arabic numerals are generally used when dealing with stages.
      ○ true
      ○ false

   4. A colon is used to express suture size, as in 7:0 Vicryl.
      ○ true
      ○ false

   5. The abbreviation AU might be mistaken for OU (each eye), so it is recommended not to use AU as an abbreviation when transcribing.
      ○ true
      ○ false

II. **MULTIPLE CHOICE.**
   Determine the correct way to transcribe each of the following.

   1. HCTZ
      ○ HCTZ
      ○ hydrochlorothiazide

   2. From 10 to 20 percent.
      ○ From 10 to 20%
      ○ From 10% to 20%

   3. The medication is to be taken q6pm.
      ○ The medication is to be taken 6 PM nightly
      ○ The medication is to be taken q.6pm.

4. The patient was born in the sixties.
   ○ The patient was born in the 60's
   ○ The patient was born in the 60s

5. She was given ten milligrams of saline.
   ○ She was given ten mg of saline
   ○ She was given 10 mg of saline

Lab Values

Numbers are used to express lab values. There are some specifics to keep in mind within the guidelines being outlined here:

Commas are NOT to be used to separate lab values from the actual test. For example: *red blood cells 400* and not *red blood cells, 400.*

Multiple lab test results are to be separated by commas if they are related. Use semicolons if the series already has internal commas. For example: *Her pH was 7.4, specific gravity 1.025, and ketones were low.*

Unrelated tests get separated by periods.

When H and H is dictated, translate to hemoglobin and hematocrit for clarity.

Specific gravity is a value associated with urine and is expressed with four digits and a decimal point, as in:

Dictated: *The specific gravity was ten thirty.*

Transcribed: *The specific gravity was 1.030.*

Headings

There are acceptable variations in terms of how the headings and subheadings of a medical report are designed and set up; however, with regard to the formatting of those particular headings, BOS instructs that "institutional and client preferences should prevail." With this in mind, some variations in formatting headings and subheadings will be outlined in this section.

Some of the variations in capitalizing headings and subheadings are as follows:

LUNGS: Within normal limits.
or
Lungs: Within normal limits.
or
Lungs
Within normal limits.
or
LUNGS
Within normal limits.

In addition to the variations in capitalization, take note of the placement of the text that follows the heading as well as the colon usage. In every case, however, the first word following the heading or subheading is to be capitalized (in the above example, *Within normal limits*).

Book of Style has its own set of formatting preferences:

Capitals are to be used for all major section headings (i.e., LUNGS, CARDIOVASCULAR, etc.).

Initial capitals are to be used in subsection headings, as below:
HEENT
Eyes:
Ears:
Nose:

Each line of both headings and subheadings should end with a period unless it is the date or the name of a person as in:
SURGEON: Harold Jones, MD
SURGEON: Harold Jones, MD, and two others.

Headings that are not dictated but are obvious may be inserted and would be something contained within account specific instructions.

Abbreviations and brief forms of the words are not to be used in headings, unless the heading is commonly done this way, as in HEENT.

Most headings are to be listed vertically and without underlining, unless specified by the client.

One exception to capitalizing the first word after the heading or subheading pertains to quantity with unit of measure, as in estimated blood loss. In a case such as this, numerals are preferred as in:
ESTIMATED BLOOD LOSS: 5 mL.

Review: Lab Values and Headings

I. **TRANSCRIPTION.**
   Edit the following dictated statements to make them compliant with the BOS style.

   1. Dictated: The H and H were 12 and 36, respectively.

   2. Dictated: Cardiovascular: regular rate and rhythm.

   3. Dictated: Specific gravity was 1018.

   4. Dictated: His lab results revealed a ph of 7 point 1 and protein of 7 milligrams per deciliter.

   5. Dictated: heent

Contractions and Hyphens

Contractions

Contractions should not be used unless they are a part of a direct quotation. In addition, abbreviations that contain contractions should be expanded. For example:

Dictated	Transcribed
won't	will not
he's	he is
it's	it is
OD'd	overdosed

Hyphenation

Both English and medical dictionaries should be consulted for proper hyphen use, but some general rules to remember follow:

Hyphens should be used to clarify meaning in certain words, such as *re-create* (to make again) instead of *recreate* (play) or *re-cover* (to cover again) and not *recover* (from an illness).

Use hyphens for pronunciation assistance as in: *co-workers* or *re-study*.

Use a hyphen when "numbers are used with words as compound modifiers preceding nouns." Examples of this are:

A 2-cm mass
The 10-mm cyst
A 6-cm incision

Suspensive hyphens are used to connect compound modifiers with the same base term as in:

The 2- and 3-mm growths
4- and 5-inch gauze

Use a hyphen when an adjective or participle is coupled with an adverb to form a compound modifier IF they precede the modifying noun but not if they follow it, as in:

A well-developed and well-nourished male patient.
versus
A male patient who is well developed and well nourished.

If an adverb ends in -ly, a hyphen should not be used when linking with a participle or adjective, as in *moderately severe pain* or *recently completed blood tests*.

The words high and low are usually hyphenated in most cases of compound adjectives, as in *low-frequency waves* or *high-density lesion*.

Numerals with words: If a number and a word form a compound modifier before a noun, it should be hyphenated as in: *2-week history* or *7-pound 3-ounce infant*.

For clarity, a hyphen is sometimes used, as in *small-bowel injury*, meaning an injury to the small bowel and not a small injury of the bowel.

Specialties: Some medical specialties, such as cardiology, use a hyphen when a term is used as an adjective, as in:

ST-T elevation
T-wave abnormality
Q-wave inversion

Genus and Species

The **genus** name is always capitalized when accompanied by the **species** name. In addition, abbreviated forms of the genus name are capitalized when accompanied by the species name. Examples are:

- Escherichia coli
- S. aureus

However, genus names should be in lowercase when used in the plural or adjectival form (or in the vernacular usage of the genus). Examples are:

- staphylococcus
- group B strep
- strep throat

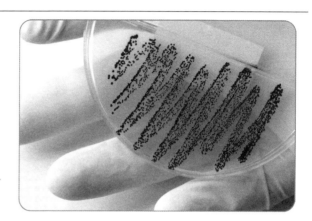

A positive lab test for staphylococcus.

Review: Contractions, Hyphens, Genus, and Species

I. **TRUE/FALSE.**
   The following are punctuated correctly: true or false?

   1. A 4 week history of pain.
      ○ true
      ○ false

   2. His large-bowel injury.
      ○ true
      ○ false

   3. The patient stated, "You won't be able to help me today."
      ○ true
      ○ false

   4. The doctor couldnt see the patient this afternoon.
      ○ true
      ○ false

5. She is a young, well-appearing, healthy female.

   ◯ true
   ◯ false

6. The patient is young, well-appearing, and healthy.

   ◯ true
   ◯ false

7. The patient was diagnosed with e. coli.

   ◯ true
   ◯ false

8. I asked my co-workers to come with me.

   ◯ true
   ◯ false

9. The lab results showed escherichia coli.

   ◯ true
   ◯ false

10. The EKG showed a Q-wave abnormality.

    ◯ true
    ◯ false

Unit 7
Using Resources Effectively

Using Resources Effectively – Introduction

Throughout your studies you will come to realize that resources are very important tools for being an accurate and productive MT (if you have not already realized that). Below is a list of some of the resources that you have at your fingertips. Just like any other tool you may have around your house or in your shed, if you don't use it you will not reap the benefits of it. So be sure to make the most of what you have available to you!

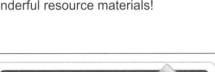

- KB BenchMark online resource – A phenomenal online resource that combines a variety of MT-specific resources into one intuitive tool.
- Career Step chat rooms, such as the medical transcription students forum and the Thursday moderated chat.
- Career Step forums – Forum boards to post questions about medications, procedures, medical terms; MT Resources Forums that provide website links, FAQs, wordlist tips, and so much more!
- "Stepping Up" newsletter – Including regular issue features that will help an MT produce accurate reports. These features include "Work Smarter, Not Harder" and "Commonly Confused Words."
- Pronunciation lists.
- Stedman's products.

Please refer to the Student Resource for more information on these wonderful resource materials!

Using Your Medical Dictionary

The best and most reliable friends you will make and keep during this program are your reference materials. In this day and age, many of your resources will be in an electronic format, although some of you may prefer to keep both online and hard-copy resources handy. Being comfortable with and using your reference materials to their fullest will make your study of terminology easier and will be excellent practice for developing practical researching skills. As far as hard-copy resources go, both the *Dorland's Medical Dictionary* and the *Stedman's Medical Dictionary* are truly remarkable resources, a marvelous reference library right at your fingertips.

Highlights

If you use your dictionary (online or hard copy) only to look up words, you are missing out on a LOT of excellent information.

To give you practice using dictionary resources, we put together some exercises. Again, these can be completed using most any type of dictionary resource—use what is comfortable to you. There may be some differences in specific definitions, but, as mentioned, the principles should be the same.

I. **MULTIPLE CHOICE.**
   Look up the following words and choose the best answer.

   chalasia

   1. The word chalasia is a (◯ noun, ◯ verb).

   2. The meaning of the original word is (◯ retrieve, ◯ relaxation).

3. Chalasia of the esophageal sphincter can cause ($\bigcirc$ vomiting, $\bigcirc$ constriction) in infants.

cirrhosis

4. The plural form of cirrhosis is ($\bigcirc$ cirrhosises, $\bigcirc$ cirrhoses, $\bigcirc$ cirrhosi).

5. The meaning of the original word is ($\bigcirc$ yellow-red, $\bigcirc$ orange-yellow).

6. Cirrhosis has reference to a disease of what organ? ($\bigcirc$ kidneys, $\bigcirc$ gallbladder, $\bigcirc$ liver)

meniscus

7. The word meniscus comes from which language? ($\bigcirc$ Latin, $\bigcirc$ Greek, $\bigcirc$ German)

8. The meaning of the original word is ($\bigcirc$ lobular, $\bigcirc$ crescent, $\bigcirc$ oval).

9. Meniscus has reference to what part of the body? ($\bigcirc$ thumb, $\bigcirc$ ankle, $\bigcirc$ knee)

pneumocrania

10. The prefix pneumo means ($\bigcirc$ head, $\bigcirc$ air, $\bigcirc$ nose).

11. Crania refers to the ($\bigcirc$ lungs, $\bigcirc$ head, $\bigcirc$ neck).

NOTE: This term does not mean "airhead" except in the most literal sense!

bezoar

12. The language from which this word comes is ($\bigcirc$ Latin, $\bigcirc$ Arabic, $\bigcirc$ Greek).

13. A bezoar is ($\bigcirc$ foreign material in the GI tract, $\bigcirc$ an abscess).

kwashiorkor

14. This word is borrowed from the language of what country? ($\bigcirc$ Egypt, $\bigcirc$ Ghana, $\bigcirc$ China)

15. Kwashiorkor is characterized by ($\bigcirc$ a deficiency in potassium and calcium, $\bigcirc$ a deficiency of calories and protein).

16. Another characteristic of this disease process is ($\bigcirc$ retarded growth, $\bigcirc$ hyperactivity).

matrix

17. The plural form of matrix is ($\bigcirc$ matrices, $\bigcirc$ matrix).

18. Matrix is ($\bigcirc$ a long-necked vessel, $\bigcirc$ tissue from which a structure develops).

Billroth or **Billroth's operation**

19. The body system on which a Billroth operation is performed (◯ GI, ◯ renal, ◯ pulmonary).

20. The procedure is also known as a (◯ colectomy, ◯ gastrectomy, ◯ pulmonectomy).

glomerulus

21. The word glomerulus is a (◯ noun, ◯ verb)

22. The plural form of the word is (◯ glomeruli, ◯ glomerulous).

23. A renal glomerulus is found within which body structure? (◯ liver, ◯ spleen, ◯ kidney).

There's A Medical Word For It

Part of the fun of learning medical terminology is discovering that there is a medical word for everything! This may be quite astonishing to you as you begin to learn the lexicon. Medical vocabulary can enliven a conversation, brighten up a cocktail party, provide around-the-dinner-table entertainment, and otherwise add a little pizazz to your day. Watch for such words, too, in your favorite novels or on your favorite TV shows. Here are a few common (and perhaps not so common) medical terms for ordinary things that you may (or may not) run into during the program or in the workplace. Below is a list of numbered terms followed by an alpha list. Fill in the blank with the best option from the alpha list and see how you do. By all means, use your medical dictionary (online or hard copy, if you have one).

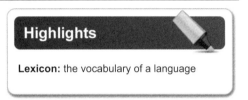

Highlights

Lexicon: the vocabulary of a language

I. MATCHING.
Match the medical term to the common term.

1. ____ acneiform pustule
2. ____ alopecia
3. ____ cephalgia
4. ____ calcaneus
5. ____ calor
6. ____ deglutition
7. ____ epistaxis
8. ____ eructation
9. ____ esotropic
10. ____ extremity
11. ____ hordeolum
12. ____ ichthyosis
13. ____ lentigo simplex
14. ____ lingua
15. ____ micturition
16. ____ nares
17. ____ omphalus
18. ____ palpebra
19. ____ phalanges
20. ____ ptarmus
21. ____ rubor
22. ____ tinea pedis
23. ____ trichobezoar
24. ____ tumor
25. ____ verruca vulgaris

A. wart
B. heat
C. hairball
D. urination
E. belly button
F. fingers and toes
G. swallowing
H. redness
I. nosebleed
J. sneezing
K. athlete's foot
L. swelling
M. stye
N. baldness
O. cross-eyed
P. headache
Q. arm or leg
R. tongue
S. belching
T. dry, scaly skin
U. freckles
V. pimple
W. heel
X. eyelid
Y. nostrils

Let Your Fingers Do the Walking

During your training, you will be challenged to research many terms and concepts.

Many of these research challenges will be found in a medical dictionary, but some you will not easily find in any hard copy dictionary. In addition, the dictionary will probably contain minimal information about them. You could go to a library, but this approach is not always practical when you are studying at home or looking for information at work!

This lesson will introduce you to some Internet **search engines and web pages** and will instruct you in making them work for you. If you are already an expert in these matters, just skip over the search instructions and go straight to the challenge words.

Keep in mind that Internet resources often need to be crosschecked for accuracy against good printed resources since sometimes there are mistakes or inconsistencies found.

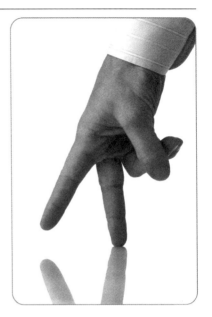

Google Search Engine

A favorite search engine for Internet users is Google. If you are not familiar with Google, you can locate it by entering http://www.google.com into your browser location bar. This search engine is very fast and easy to use.

You may want to bookmark Google, as you will most likely refer to it frequently both throughout this training program and once working as an MT.

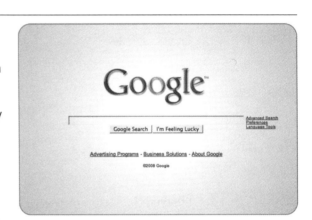

How To Search

To search in Google, just type in a few descriptive words into the search bar and click the Google search button for a list of results. Google will search for pages that match your search terms, so if you can not find what you are looking for—try using different variations of your search terms.

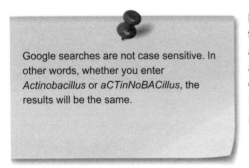

Google searches are not case sensitive. In other words, whether you enter *Actinobacillus* or *aCTinNoBACillus*, the results will be the same.

For example, if a search for *incus* (a small bone in the ear) didn't turn up what you were looking for, you could try adding a few additional keywords such as *incus ear anatomy*. Sometimes just adding the name of the specialty, in this case otology or otorhinolaryngology, will produce better results. Other words that may be helpful in narrowing a search are *medical*, *clinical*, *patient*, *glossary*, or *surgery*.

Career Step is not affiliated with Google. Google.com is just one of many good sources available and is used here for illustrative purposes.

Narrowing Your Google Search

Quotation Marks, Plus Sign, and Minus Sign

Quotation Marks – Using quotation marks will create a phrase, and Google will search for that phrase exactly as you typed it. For example, entering "pulmonary thrombus" (with the quotation marks) will show results with terms appearing in that exact order.

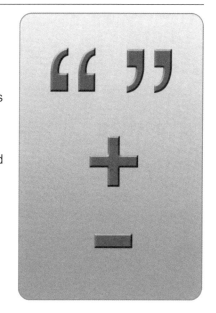

Plus Sign – Google will ignore certain common words such as *and*, *is*, and *how*. It will also ignore some single digits and single letters. If the word is important to your search, use the plus sign before the word. Be sure to add a space before the + symbol. Google will ignore the *and* unless you enter the plus sign in front of it. For example, If you are searching for the phras *incus and stapes* and need to have it appear in that order, you will need to enter *incus +and stapes* into the search box.

Minus Sign – The minus sign will eliminate any result with that word. For example, if you want to find pages on encephalopathy, but not on bovine spongiform encephalopathy, you will need to enter *encephalopathy - bovine -spongiform*. Remember to put a space before the minus sign.

Advanced Search

Google, like most search engines, allows you to perform an **Advanced Search** (just click the advanced search link). This allows you to put very specific guidelines into your search. You will see some of the same search features we just discussed, such as using an exact phrase or omitting a certain word from your search. But there are other features as well that might be new to you:

- one or more of these words
- file type
- how recent the page is (you may need to click on the *Date*, *Usage Rights*, *Numeric Range*, and *More* link to expand this feature).

Highlight Your Results

Google offers a great feature called the cache link. For example, let's say you are searching for information on pulmonary thrombus. Underneath each of the results is a cache link.

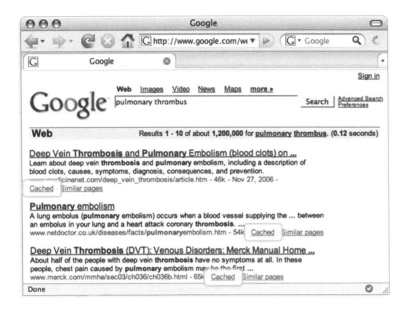

Clicking on these cache links will return pages with the keywords highlighted within that document. Each keyword is assigned a different color. This is a helpful feature that enables you to quickly scroll the document to find what you are looking for.

On occasion you will find that a site does not provide a cache link or that using the cache link changes the formatting of the site so that it is not easily read. Your computer's *Find* feature will also work on websites (Ctrl + f).

Career Step is not affiliated with Google. Google.com is just one of many good sources available and is used here for illustrative purposes.

Getting More Out of Google

Making Google Yours

Google can be customized in a number of ways:

- search only for pages in English
- use different levels of filtering
- display 10 to 100 results per page
- open results in a new or same browser window

Simply click on *preferences* on Google's home page to adjust any of these customizations. Be sure to click on *Save Preferences* on the bottom right of the page or else your preferences will be set back to default the next time you visit the Google page.

Finding Definitions

Google also provides a link for dictionary definitions served by Answers.com.

This is a very useful feature. To try this out do a search for the word *xanthosis*. Now check the results message that appears above and to the right of the search results. The results message shows how many pages were found for your search. For example, the results message for the "xanthosis" search says: Results 1-10 of about 6,860 (this is probably more today…it grows daily!) English pages for xanthosis [definition].

In the results message, xanthosis is followed by [definition], which is underlined. This is a clickable link. Select this link and the Answers.com definition will be displayed. This is a great feature and you might find it very useful to help you in your studies.

Google Images

Sometimes seeing what you're searching for is more helpful than reading about it. For example, it might be hard to imagine the location of a certain ligament if it is being described in words such as *anterior to this but posterior to that*. But if you could just **see** where it is located in relation to other structures, it would be much easier to envision it yourself. Or sometimes seeing what a piece of surgical equipment looks like helps you better imagine how it is used than reading a detailed sentence about it. In these instances, just click on the Images link in the top right corner of Google. I mean really—who knew a Kerrison rongeur looked like this?

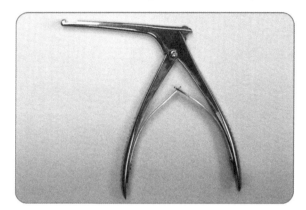

Google Images did, that's who!

Google, of course, is not the only search engine for medical subjects. The general principles for searching Google can also be used on other web sites. It would benefit you to become familiar with the sites listed in the following pages of this unit.

Career Step is not affiliated with Google. Google.com is just one of many good sources available and is used here for illustrative purposes.

Review: Google

I. **TRUE/FALSE.**
   Mark the following true or false.

   1. Google searches are case sensitive.

      ◯ true
      ◯ false

   2. A cache link is a good way to easily locate a keyword on a website.

      ◯ true
      ◯ false

3. You can customize Google to only display English language pages.
   ○ true
   ○ false

4. Using quotation marks around a phrase will allow you to eliminate that phrase from your search results, thus narrowing your results.
   ○ true
   ○ false

5. Google provides a definition link in the results message, but you have to include the term *definition* in your search for this link to appear.
   ○ true
   ○ false

II. MATCHING.
Match the correct term to the definition.

1. ____ Allows you to create saved search settings.
2. ____ Omits the word from your search.
3. ____ A comprehensive definition site.
4. ____ Allows you to create a very specific search.
5. ____ Requires the word be included in your search.
6. ____ A search engine.

A. Plus sign
B. Answers.com
C. Google.com
D. Preferences
E. Minus sign
F. Advanced search

Additional Helpful Sites

There are scores and scores of additional helpful websites for researching medical information. Here are a handful:

http://www.onelook.com – Dictionary that allows you to search in other dictionaries, all at one time. This is especially helpful if you have difficulty finding a given definition. Like Google, it has different features for searching, such as using * for a fuzzy search. This feature can save your sanity when trying to figure out the spelling of a word!

http://www.media4u.com/bbp/medabb_a.html – Medical abbreviation site that has several thousand entries.

http://http://www.medilexicon.com/ – Medical abbreviations, dictionaries, news, and pharmacology site.

http://www.renesue.com – A home page created by a CS graduate, it contains dozens of good MT links. If the number of links is overwhelming, you might want to start by checking out the links under MT References.

http://www.dailygrammar.com – Grammar site that is helpful to have on hand, especially if grammar is giving you fits.

The possibilities are truly limitless. Some of these sites may become your favorites. You may discover favorites of your own. In any case, wherever you go with your medical language training, the Internet is an inexhaustible resource.

Resource Challenge

Okay, are you ready for a challenge? See if you can search the web to find definitions for the following terms. It may be that some of them can be found in a medical dictionary. For this exercise we want you to leave any hard copy dictionaries closed! Sit on them if you have to—this is an exercise in using Internet resources!

- Christmas disease
- fetal warfarin syndrome
- collyrium
- subarachnoid cistern
- bovarism
- Einthoven's triangle

Use the techniques discussed above to research these terms. Note the results, and then complete the exercise below.

I. **MATCHING.**
   Match the correct term to the definition.

1. ___ Eyewash.

2. ___ A form of hemophilia.

3. ___ Standard electrocardiogram lead points.

4. ___ Excessive and unwarranted self estimate.

5. ___ A structure in the brain.

6. ___ Drug-induced birth defects.

A. Christmas disease
B. bovarism
C. fetal warfarin syndrome
D. collyrium
E. Einthoven's triangle
F. subarachnoid cistern

Check Your Research

Christmas disease: Christmas disease is one of the two main forms of hemophilia and is sometimes called hemophilia B. Guess what the other type is called. You're right. Hemophilia A. Hemophilia accounts for 90 percent of such hereditary bleeding disorders, while the more rare Christmas disease afflicts about 10 percentof hemophilia patients.

Both Christmas disease and hemophilia A are genetic disorders in which there is deficient production of one of the proteins in the blood. Individuals with Christmas disease have a deficiency in a protein called factor IX, while in hemophilia A the deficiency is factor VIII. Patients lacking these proteins take longer to form blood clots, and prolonged bleeding can occur after a cut or bruise.

The disease was named fairly recently, in 1952, after a man named Stephen Christmas, who was the first patient proven to have the disorder.

Hemophilia is historically important, having afflicted many of the male descendants of Queen Victoria, including Alexei, the son of the last Russian Czar. He was murdered along with his four sisters and his mother and father at the time of the Russian Revolution. Some historians have argued that if Alexei had not had hemophilia, there would never have been a Russian Revolution. But who can say?

fetal warfarin syndrome: Coumarins can cross the placenta to the fetus, which is highly sensitive to them. Fetal warfarin syndrome may occur in up to 25% of fetuses exposed to warfarin during the 1st trimester. Abnormalities include nasal hypoplasia, bone stippling (seen on x-rays), bilateral optic atrophy, and various degrees of mental retardation. Exposure to warfarin during the 2nd or 3rd trimester has been related to optic atrophy, cataracts, mental retardation, microcephaly, and microphthalmia.

As you see, there are some really good medical words to add to your notebook in the above definition. In fact, the definition won't make any sense to you if you don't know the meaning of *coumarin, warfarin, hypoplasia, atrophy, microcephaly,* and *microphthalmia.*

collyrium: A medicinal lotion applied to the eye (eyewash). This is not a brand name, but a word that describes any such salve or lotion. The plural form is collyria.

subarachnoid cistern The subarachnoid cistern is a sac or cavity of the subarachnoid space that contains cerebrospinal fluid. This is a part of the central nervous system structure between the lower brain and upper spinal cord.

subarachnoid: situated or occurring beneath the arachnoid membrane, or between the arachnoid and the pia mater.

cistern: a sac or cavity containing fluid, especially lymph or cerebrospinal fluid. This is, of course, the anatomical definition. Cistern also has a broader, more general meaning.

bovarism: bovarism (n.) BO-vuh-rizm 1. an exaggerated, especially glamorized, estimate of oneself; conceit. The term comes from literature, specifically from the novel *Madame Bovary*, by the great French novelist, Gustave Flaubert. To the bovarist, the gap between the overblown self-perception and the actual reality leads to irreconcilable personality conflict.

Do you know anybody like that?

Einthoven's triangle: An imaginary equilateral triangle with the heart at its center and representing the three standard limb leads of the electrocardiogram when the apex is at the pelvis. This is named after William Einthoven, a Dutch doctor who developed the first electrocardiograph, or EKG.

How to Look up Words

Being able to effectively look up words is of utmost importance. As a medical transcriptionist, you need to have both an understanding of the words used and be able to correctly spell them! While the Internet is a wonderful resource, be aware that not all sites are error-free or even pay attention to spelling to begin with! Therefore, it is very important to double-check spelling and not just go with a spelling because it rendered in the search results. Doing so can cost you valuable points on the final exam and employment tests and can affect the meaning of a medical report or make it too difficult to understand.

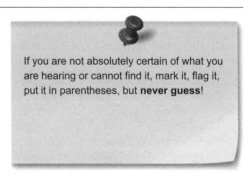

If you are not absolutely certain of what you are hearing or cannot find it, mark it, flag it, put it in parentheses, but **never guess**!

When transcribing you will hear a lot of words that you don't know. Consequently, you will need to have reference books and know how to use them. **Do not guess**. I cannot emphasize the importance of this enough. **Never** guess. A medical report is a legal document and should be treated as such—with careful attention to detail. It is important that you transcribe exactly what the dictator says (with the exception of ensuring grammatical correctness). Guessing about the spelling of a word can change the meaning of the sentence or render it totally meaningless, thus compromising the entire report.

In order to find words you hear or verify terms you read, you must know how to look up words. Presumably, the information covered so far in this unit will make looking up words much easier for you, but there are helpful hints you can utilize to make locating a new word easier.

Silent First Characters

First of all, in order to even begin looking up a word, you must be able to identify what the initial sound(s) is (are). Obviously, it is impossible to start with the letter *A* and go through the entire dictionary looking for a word if you have no idea what it begins with. However, there are several different scenarios that make it difficult to determine correctly which letter to look under.

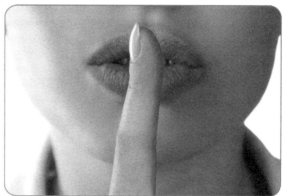

The first of these is silent letters. The most common example of this is found in words like *knife* and *knee*. Although the word begins with the letter *K*, the initial SOUND is "N". Therefore, even if you were correctly able to determine that it started with an "N" sound, you would never locate the correct word by looking only under the letter *N*. You should keep *K* in mind when searching for any word beginning with an "N" sound that you cannot find under *N*.

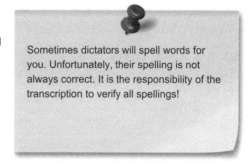

Sometimes dictators will spell words for you. Unfortunately, their spelling is not always correct. It is the responsibility of the transcription to verify all spellings!

There is another letter that is often silent in medical words. However, this letter can be placed in front of four different consonants. The letter is *P*. It is silent in the words *pneumonia* and *pneumothorax* (giving the initial sound "N"). It is also silent in the words *psoas* and *psoriasis* (giving the initial sound "S"). It is silent in the words *pterygium* and *ptosis* (giving the initial sound "T").

Finally, it is silent in the word *Pfannenstiel* (giving an initial sound of "F"). Clearly, these words would be difficult or impossible to locate if you did not know that they began with the letter *P*. If you are having trouble locating a word with the initial sound of "S," "T," or "N," try searching for it in the *P* section of the dictionary. These are examples only, and there are multiple instances of words like these.

Another silent letter that can confuse the process of looking up a word is the letter *H*. It is often silent when placed next to an *R*. Specifically, the words *rheumatoid, rhinitis, rhinoplasty, rhabdomyolysis*, and *rhonchi* are not found under *R* plus a vowel. Therefore, when searching for letters with the initial sound "R" remember to try looking under *RH*.

Silent letters present the biggest problem when determining where to begin your search. However, the longer a word gets, the more you need to be aware of alternative spellings. Therefore, correctly determining what letter your word begins with is a great place to start, but you need to know more, and silent letters are not the only things confounding your search. In the English language several sounds are represented by different letters or groups of letters. The most basic of these were learned in elementary school—an "S" sound, which can be written with an *S*, as in *slide* or with a *C*, as in *city*. The greater variety of spelling possibilities you master for a particular sound, the more equipped you are to locate an unfamiliar word in the dictionary. Following are a number of sounds and the different consonant combinations that can make them.

The group of letters that make up the sound is capitalized in the sample words. Of course, these lists are samples only and are by no means exhaustive.

Sound: S as in *Side*

Some possible letter combinations that make this sound are: S, C, SC, SCH

aCephaly	calCific	Cecal
baCillus	Cephalad	Cerumen
CeSarean	Cicatrix	deCidua
ESCHerichia	oSCillating	faCet
faSCicular	Sideroblast	

Sound: F as in *Fly*

Some possible letter combinations that make this sound are: F, PH

apoPHysis	asPHyxia	aPHagia
PHosPHatase	emPHysema	Frenulum
egoPHony	Facet	PHlebolith

Sound: K as in *Kiss*

Some possible letter combinations that make this sound are: CH, C, K, CCH, QU

aCHalasia	araCHnoid	braCHium
caCHexia	Coccyx	CHlamydia
anKylosing	eCCHymosis	MCIvor
teCHniQUe	iCHthyosis	Keloid
aCrodynia	Condylar	opaQUe

Sound: Z as in *Zebra*

Some possible letter combinations that make this sound are: Z, S, X

aZotemia	peS	Xanthoma
moSaiciSm	Xerostomia	roSacea
eXanthem	Zygoma	

Sound: CH as in *Church*

Some possible letter combinations that make this sound are: CH, T, TCH, CT

boTulism	stiTCH	CHamfer
muCH	CephalpaTulous	piCTure

Sound: ZH as in *Pleasure*

Some possible letter combinations that make this sound are: G, DJ, DG, S

bouGie	aDJuvant	pleDGet
albuGinea	torSion	lavaGe

Sound: SH as in *Push*

Some possible letter combinations that make this sound are: C, CH, SC, SCH, SH

alopeCia	dystoCia	eustaCHian
faSCia	SCHwannoma	rosaCea
sebaCeous	SHelf	waSH

Enunciation

Another problem you will come across in transcription is that some letters that are quite different if enunciated carefully, sound exactly the same when spoken quickly in a sentence. A good example of this includes the sounds "T" and "D." Clearly, you can understand the difference when spoken slowly and carefully. However, say the word *batter* quickly. If you didn't know that there were two *T*'s in this word, it would be difficult to tell if it required a *T* or a *D*. A couple of medical examples of this are *aditus* and *tardive*. If you come across a sound in transcription that cannot clearly be distinguished as a "T" or a "D," check under both letters.

You can further increase your chances of locating a difficult word if you take into consideration that it could contain double consonants. You have already seen examples of this in the Medical Word Building module of this course. Remember, the suffix for excessive flow or discharge is -rrhagia. There are others that contain two *R*'s. Some other examples are *dissemination*, *tinnitus*, *sagittal*, *vaccinate*, and *coccyx*. In looking up words, keep double consonants in mind as an alternative.

Another source of confusion in medical reports is the use of foreign terms. Unless you are knowledgeable in another language, it will be difficult for you to locate these. I have included the most common ones and their pronunciations.

1. en bloc (pronounced on block).
2. bruit(s) (pronounced broo-ee in both singular and plural)
3. raphe (pronounced rafay)
4. rales* (pronounced ralz—as in cat)
5. Virchow-Robin (pronounced verkow roban)
6. Gilbert's disease (pronouonced zhee-bears)
7. peau d'orange (pronounced po-d'ranzh)
8. Raynaud disease (pronounced rayno)

You will also hear this pronounced "rails," and "rawls ."

One of the greatest difficulties encountered in locating an unknown word in the dictionary is determining which vowels are being said. While it is easy to mistake consonants for each other when they are spoken quickly, it is even worse with vowels. When said fast, just about any vowel can be mistaken for almost any other, and when you add difficult medical spellings, it is even worse. Be sure to always check all possible vowels in a word before giving up. Following are some of the more common vowel combinations and the sounds they make.

Perhaps the most confusing vowel, which appears quite often in medical reports, is *Y*. It can have several different sounds and, at least at first, it may not occur to a new transcriptionist to look for it. Pay careful attention to the *Y* and the possible sounds it can have.

Sound: I as in *Pig*

mYdriasis	mYxoid	sYnchondrosis
sYnechia	polYp	sYlvian
spondYlolysis	dIpsia	dYspnea
dYsEntery	dIssemInation	dYstocia

Sound: U as in *You*

EUstachian	EUthyroid	EUkaryon

Sound: I as in *Light*

mYositis	mYelitis	nYstagmus
odYnophagia	lEIomYoma	sIte
REIter's	lIGHt	strIdor

Sound: EU as in *Nerve*

nEUroma   plEUrisy   anEUrysm

Sound: UH as in *Mud*

labYrinth   anAphYlaxis   metaphYsis
blOOd   epiphYsis   deciduA
bacillUs   azygOUs   cecAl

Sound: EE as in *Street*

pYriform   Iglesias   synEchia
ErythEma   libIdo   biopsY

Sound: A as in *Play*

IglEsias   parEnchyma   Ankylosing

Sound: OO as in *Food*

OOphorectomy   pUdendal   manEUver

Sound: A as in *Cat*

grAAfian   metAphysis   lAbyrinth
Aneurysm   Asphyxia   vAstus

Sound: E as in *Hen*

rOEntgEnogram   Erythema   cachExia
erythEmatous   lIbido   myElination

Sound: AH as in *Ma*

pOlyp   spOndylosis   jAUndice
cOccyx   amAUrosis   AUricular

I. **TRUE/FALSE.**
    Mark the following true or false.

1. The word *dysentery* rhymes with the word *missionary*.

    ○ true
    ○ false

2. The word *Reiter's* rhymes with the word *feeders*.

    ○ true
    ○ false

3. The word *cecal* rhymes with the word *fecal*.

    ○ true
    ○ false

120

4. The word *libido* rhymes with the word *tuxedo*.

   ○ true
   ○ false

5. The word *polyp* rhymes with the word *wallop*.

   ○ true
   ○ false

Context Clues

There is another method of looking up words that will make your transition into transcription much easier. Some medical words you will never find if you simply look for them in the dictionary under the initial sound. An example is the term *Burkitt's*. It is not found under *B*. You should make it a habit, before you begin looking in the dictionary, to notice the word immediately FOLLOWING or PRECEDING the one you are looking for. Burkitt's would not be dictated by itself. It would be in a sentence or a diagnosis list like "Burkitt's lymphoma." Listed under *lymphoma* in the dictionary is a whole series of words in alphabetical order. Several such general words appear in the dictionary with lists categorized alphabetically under them representing specific types. Following are some of them. Keep in mind that if you cannot locate a word, and you have tried all reasonable letter combinations, it could be found under the word that immediately precedes or follows it.

Again, this is only a PARTIAL list. A term, for example, like *cirrhosis*, represents a disease that can take several forms or have several varieties, all of which might be listed in the dictionary under *cirrhosis*: acute juvenile cirrhosis, Laennec's cirrhosis, syphilitic cirrhosis, and others. Knowing this shortcut can potentially save you much time and frustration. Note that many of the words on this list are surgical instruments and can be found in a good surgical word book.

ACID	FRACTURE	OSTEOTOME
ALOPECIA	GAG	PACEMAKER
ANESTHESIA	GAIT	PIN
ARTERY	GAUZE	PLATE
BAG	GLAND	POSITION
BANDAGE	GOUGE	PROCEDURE
BRACE	GRAFT	PROSTHESIS
CANAL	HOOK	PSYCHOSIS
CATHETER	IMPLANT	RASP
CAUTERY	INCISION	REAMER
CELL	KERATITIS	REFLEX
CIRRHOSIS	KNIFE	RETRACTOR
CLAMP	LENS	RONGEUR
CONDITION	LIGAMENT	SAW
CURET	LINE	SCISSORS
CYST	LINEA	SCREW
DEFORMITY	MANEUVER	SHEATH
DERMATITIS	MURMUR	SHIELD
DISEASE	MUSCLE	SIGN
DRESSING	NAIL	SNARE
ELEVATOR	NEEDLE	SPECULUM
EPILEPSY	NEPHRITIS	SPLINT
FILAMENT	NERVE	STAIN
FILTER	NODE	SUTURE
FORCEPS	OPERATION	

Phonetics (Fuh-net-icks)

While phonetic charts can sometimes be confusing, they are also a great resource once you figure out how to read them. In this chart, the letter or combination of letters on the left makes the sound in bold in the familiar word to the right. For quick reference, this chart is broken down into consonants and vowels.

CONSONANTS
b – Boat
k – Cat
d – Dog
f – Fun
g – Game
h – Hi
j – Jump
l – Love
m – Mine
n – Nice
p – Pet
r – Run
s – Save
v – Vine
w – Way
y – Yellow
z – jaZZ
ch – CHurCH
sh – SHow
th – THink

VOWELS
A – mAke
ah – tAll
a – cAt
E – sEAl
e – rEd
I – slIde
i – sIt
O – bOAt
oo – yOU
u – mUd

You may need to use a dictionary, or a handy-dandy Internet site like www.onelook.com, to complete the exercises. There is at least one word spelled out phonetically in each question, and there are spaces between sounds that require two letters, such as *sh* or *ah*. Say the word aloud, find it in your resources, and enter it in the space provided.

I. FILL IN THE BLANK.
Enter the correct word in the blank provided.

1.   His alkaline (f ah sfutAs) is 12. _____

2.   His ears contained a large amount of (seroomen). _____

3.   He underwent (ajuvent) chemotherapy. _____

4.   There is evidence of a (kahlEz) fracture. _____

5.   She has a history of (roomatik) fever. _____

6.   (Surlusis) was noted. _____

7.   She was born with (p ah lEdaktulE). _____

8.   A (fanenstEl) incision was made. _____

9.   Pain was noted in the (zIfOyd) area. _____

10. The optic (klazm) is normal. _____

11. A 3-0 (vIkrul) suture was used to close the skin. _____

12. She underwent (sEk ah stumE). _____

13. A (nubO th Een) cyst was noted. _____

14. She had evidence of (grafEen) follicles. _____

15. A (rooenwI) anastomosis was accomplished. _____

16. (klipul fIl) syndrome was suspected. _____

17. The (mOyetl) was normal. _____

18. She had a (fusikyooler) block. _____

19. He had (lerinjEel) carcinoma. _____

20. There is evidence of a (sh mOrelz) node. _____

21. She has (doopetrenz) contracture. _____

22. (KrOnz) disease is the expected etiology. _____

23. A (jaksunprat) drain was inserted._____

24. There was a pectus (kArin ah tum) deformity._____

25. She underwent (fasetektuml)._____

26. The (ah sulAtEng) saw was used._____

27. There was lamina (puprE sh yu)._____

28. We used (dubAkE) forceps._____

29. There was a (n ah k sh us) odor._____

30. There was (ekimOsis) of the area._____

31. She was diagnosed with (kahapOsEz) sarcoma._____

32. He had (tinutis)._____

33. He had a (turijEum) of the left eye._____

34. There was pain in the (skafOyd) area._____

35. Culture grew out pseudomonas (OrigenOsu)._____

36. His skin was (pa ch yoolus)._____

37. He had a (pez plAnum) deformity._____

38. He had (ozgud sh l ah terz) disease._____

39. She was diagnosed with (emfuzEma)._____

40. There was a (sh w ah nOmu)._____

41. (VaksinA sh unz) are up to date._____

42. (Tinelz) sign was negative._____

43. A (sh ah tskEz) ring was noted._____

44. She had (sebOrAik) keratosis._____

45. He had right (Orikyooler) pain._____

46. The (simfusis) pubis is intact._____

47. The patient had (disna th Eyu)._____

48. A (boozhE) was used._____

49. No (perAnkimul) infiltrates. _____

50. The baby had (j ah ndis). _____

Using Resources Tips

Given these phonetic conundrums, you will be happy to know that there are also some very good tips on how to make looking up words easier!

1. Take note of the word immediately following or preceding the word you are looking for. For example, if you are looking for a certain type of prosthesis, you may have better luck finding it under the category *prosthesis* and then browsing the subcategory of types of prostheses found there. Or when using a search engine, you might find that including another appropriate word provides you with a suggested spelling. (Google will sometimes suggest a spelling if it feels your spelling may be incorrect; however, always verify the correct spelling in a reliable resource, as even Google is sometimes wrong!) An example of this might be *cruciate ligament*. Let's say you don't know the spelling of *cruciate* and your phonetic guess is *crucheat*. This alone will not bring up any results from Google. However, if you put in *crucheat ligament*, Google will suggest *cruciate ligament* as the correct spelling.

2. Make use of fuzzy searches. Onelook (www.onelook.com), among other sites, allows you to use * in place of letters you are unsure of. This includes the initial letter of a word. This can save you a lot of time if you are sure of certain parts of a word but very unsure about other parts! For instance, perhaps you are unsure of all of the vowels in *ginglymoid*. You might put *g*ngl*moid* into Onelook's search bar to find that it only comes up with one word: *ginglymoid*.

3. Narrow your search whenever possible. Features of Google that have already been discussed, such as using quotations marks and the plus and minus signs, are great time savers—when you use them! Onelook also has a time-saving feature—you can choose to narrow your search to **Common Words Only** by clicking on this selection on the upper right side. Of course, sometimes you will want to see **All Matches** and can select this feature as well. Using the same example above—*ginglymoid*—perhaps you really are unsure of the spelling because the dictator sure is mumbling! But you can come up with *gi*d*. Onelook will show you 396 (maybe more) possible results if you select **All Matches**! If you select **Common Words and Phrases Only** it will narrow your search down significantly to 60 (or so) results. However, if you click on **Common Words Only**, your search will be further narrowed down to only 33 (ish) results. Now, isn't that much better than browsing your way through 396 terms?

Review: How to Look up Words

I. TRUE/FALSE.
Mark the following true or false.

1. In the English language, all letters only have one possible pronunciation.
   ○ true
   ○ false

2. Foreign terms are sometimes used as part of medical terminology.
   ○ true
   ○ false

3. One good way to find a new word is to look it up under its category, such as disease.
   ○ true
   ○ false

4. Onelook does not allow you to use a fuzzy search.
   ○ true
   ○ false

5. The only time-saving feature on Onelook is to select All Matches.
   ○ true
   ○ false

II. FILL IN THE BLANK.
Each sentence has a word spelled phonetically. Enter the correct medical term in the blank.

1. A (fAlan) test was performed. _____

2. Single intrauterine (jestAshun) is seen. _____

3. No (ralz), rhonchi, or wheezes. _____

4. She was noted to have (kahlEz) fracture. _____

5. Her (amulAz) is within normal limits. _____

6. No spinal (hIpurtrufE). _____

7. Her (dOrsiflekshun) was normal. _____

8. A (dahplur) ultrasound was done. _____

Unit 8
Medical Ethics and Confidentiality

Medical Ethics and Confidentiality – Introduction

Much of your studies preparing you for a career as a medical transcriptionist deal with language, terminology, anatomy, and pharmacology because these are the tools you will be utilizing every day. But you should never forget that what you are really working with and working for are people. Every medical record you transcribe is a snapshot in the life of a person, often at their most vulnerable. You must remind yourself that as an MT you hold a position dealing with very powerful and personal information about people and your professional duties require you to take a conscientious and ethical approach to this material.

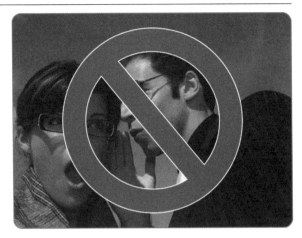

The Medical Ethics and Confidentiality unit will focus on the role of the medical transcriptionist when dealing with healthcare documentation. Professional standards, a changing healthcare information environment, and the laws and ethics governing healthcare information all play important parts in guiding an MT through his/her daily work. In an effort to be an effective and exacting MT, you will want to be sure you are familiar with and diligent in applying the rules and guidelines governing medical ethics and confidentiality.

The Need for Documentation Standards

The importance of accurate and timely medical record documentation and protecting the confidentiality of the medical record cannot be overemphasized. Why? Because behind every medical record there is a person. A real person. Here are a few scenarios to bring home the importance of accuracy, timeliness, and confidentiality:

Highlights

Behind every medical record there is a person. A real person.

Scenario 1:

Alex is scheduled to undergo a surgical procedure on her left leg. The documentation in her medical record inaccurately states the surgery is to be performed on her right leg. She is taken to the operating room where they operate on the wrong leg.

Scenario 2:

Your daughter is brought to the emergency room following an accident and is admitted to the hospital. A history is taken, including the fact that she is allergic to penicillin, but the report is not returned to the medical record for several days. Your daughter develops a dangerously high fever and is given a shot of penicillin. She goes into anaphylactic shock and comes close to death.

Scenario 3:

Kelly visits a local clinic for blood work and learns she has AIDS. The clinic's computer is "hacked" into and her personal information and AIDS status are printed on an anti-homosexual flyer in her hometown.

Each of these scenarios represents a serious breakdown in the handling of private healthcare information. As you can see, the consequences can be embarrassing, painful, and—at worst—catastrophic. Quality documentation is an important component of quality patient care. In this unit we'll take a closer look at medical records documentation standards and oversight, industry trends in medical documentation, common documentation errors, and the role medical transcriptionists play in ensuring integrity in the medical record.

Healthcare Documentation Organizations

The United States has progressed from the days of the wild West when the storekeeper could hang out a shingle in a one-horse town and say he sold chocolate bars and tobacco, cut hair, extracted teeth, and removed bullets! Today, if you want to hang out a "shingle" as a healthcare provider, your rights and responsibilities are clear. Healthcare services are regulated and can only be provided by professionals under strict state and federal guidelines. Standards for healthcare documentation are laid out by accrediting organizations and monitored by governmental and accrediting organizations.

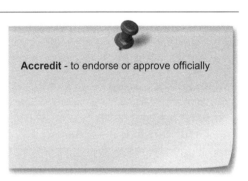

Accredit - to endorse or approve officially

In the United States, medical record documentation must be uniform, accurate, complete, legible, and timely. It is the responsibility of every healthcare professional (also known as **HIM [health information management] professional**) to be informed about healthcare documentation standards and to work with other HIM professionals to ensure accurate, timely documentation so that patients receive quality care.

Highlights

It is the responsibility of every healthcare professional (also known as **HIM [health information management] professional** to be informed about healthcare documentation standards and to work with other HIM professionals to ensure accurate, timely documentation so that patients receive quality care.

Several organizations have developed medical record documentation standards. One such organization is The Joint Commission. This organization accredits the majority of U.S. hospitals and other healthcare organizations. In addition to The Joint Commission, here is a partial list of organizations that have established documentation standards:

- National Committee for Quality Assurance (NCQA)
- American Accreditation Healthcare Commission/Utilization Review Accreditation Commission (AAHCC/URAC)
- American Osteopathic Association (AOA)
- Commission on Accreditation of Rehabilitation Facilities (CARF)
- Health Accreditation Program of the National League of Nursing
- College of American Pathologists (CAP)
- American Association of Blood Banks (AABB)
- American College of Surgeons (ACS)
- Accreditation Association for Ambulatory Healthcare (AAAHC)
- American Medical Accreditation Program (AMAP)
- American Health Information Management Association (AHIMA)

Depending on where your career path takes you and what type of healthcare provider employs you, you will be involved with one or more of these organizations. It is essential that HIM professionals become familiar with the standards and documentation requirements of the organizations which provide oversight to their employer. Documentation standards change from year to year. Medical transcriptionists need to stay abreast of updates and changes so they can assure ongoing quality patient care.

Documentation Standards

Documentation standards are developed by different organizations to ensure the uniformity, accuracy, completeness, legibility, authenticity, frequency, and format of medical record entries.

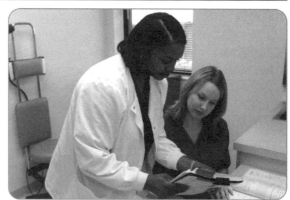

As mentioned on the previous page, many organizations provide **documentation standards** and oversight. The American Health Information Management Association (AHIMA) has developed general documentation standards/guidelines to ensure patients receive quality care. We'll use the AHIMA standards as an example.

The guidelines developed by AHIMA include the following:

Standard 1: Every healthcare organization should have policies that ensure the uniformity of both the content and the format of the medical record. The policies should be based on all applicable accreditation standards, federal and state regulations, payer requirements, and professional practice standards.

Standard 2: The medical record should be organized systematically in order to facilitate data retrieval and compilation.

Standard 3: Only individuals authorized by the organization's policies should be allowed to enter documentation in the medical record.

Standard 4: Organizational policy and/or the medical staff rules and regulations should specify who may receive and transcribe verbal physician's orders.

Standard 5: Medical record entries should be documented at the time that the services they describe are rendered.

Standard 6: The authors of all entries should be clearly identified in the record.

Standard 7: Only abbreviations and symbols approved by the organization and/or medical staff rules and regulations should be used in the medical record.

Standard 8: All entries in the medical record should be permanent.

> **Highlights**
>
> **Definition:**
> **Qualitative analysis:** Review of the medical record to ensure that standards are met and to determine accuracy of record documentation.
> **Quantitative analysis:** Review of the medical record to determine its completeness.

Standard 9: Errors in paper-based records should be corrected according to the following process: Draw a single line in ink through the incorrect entry. Then print the word error at the top of the entry along with a legal signature or initials and the date, time, and reason for change and the title and discipline of the individual making the correction. The correct information is then added to the entry. Errors may never be obliterated. The original entry should remain legible, and the corrections should be entered in chronological order. Any late entries should be labeled as such. Similar requirements apply to computer-based records.

Standard 10: Any corrections or information added to the record by the patient should be inserted as an addendum. No changes should be made in the original entries in the record. Any information added to the medical record by the patient should be clearly identified as an addendum.

Standard 11: The health information department (medical records) should develop, implement, and evaluate policies and procedures related to the qualitative and quantitative analysis of medical records.

With these standards in mind, let's look at two important definitions:

Acceptable documentation – documentation (a medical record) that conforms to documentation standards by presenting an accurate, complete, legible, chronological account of the care provided to the patient.

Unacceptable documentation – documentation that does **not** conform to documentation standards—it is somehow unclear, incomplete, or inaccurate.

I. **MULTIPLE CHOICE.**
Document Analysis. Using the AHIMA documentation standards listed above, read each example and determine if the documentation sample or practice is acceptable documentation or unacceptable documentation.

> **Standard 9**: Errors in paper-based records should be corrected according to the following process: Draw a single line in ink through the incorrect entry. Then print the word error at the top of the entry along with a legal signature or initials and the date, time, and reason for change and the title and discipline of the individual making the correction. The correct information is then added to the entry. Errors may never be obliterated. The original entry should remain legible, and the corrections should be entered in chronological order. Any late entries should be labeled as such. Similar requirements apply to computer-based records.

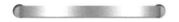

Medical Record

DIAGNOSIS: Degenerative joint disease lumbar spine.

MP 10-17-06
PROCEDURE: Facet joint injection, L4-L5 ~~and L3-L4,~~ both sides.

The patient was placed in the prone position on the x-ray table. He was monitored by O2 saturation, pulse, blood pressure, and EKG and was given 100 mcg of Fentanyl and 8 mg of Versed. Under fluoroscopy, a spinal needle was inserted down at the level of the facet joint on left side and was injected with approximately 1 cc of Kenalog and a local anesthetic solution comprised of 1% Xylocaine and 40 mg of Kenalog in the total dosage. The patient tolerated the procedure well and was returned to the ASU for postoperative care.

1. While reviewing the procedure note of Jane Smith*, Dr. Jones realized that the procedure was carried out on L4-L5 but not on L3-L4. He marked through the erroneous information and initialed and dated the error.
   - ⚪ acceptable documentation
   - ⚪ unacceptable documentation

Name changed to protect confidentiality.

> **Standard 5**: Medical record entries should be documented at the time that the services they describe are rendered.

2. Jack is taken in for surgery on October 11. He visits the physical therapist to begin physical therapy on October 19. The operative report is not available for the physical therapist to review because the surgeon has not yet dictated the report.
   - ⚪ acceptable documentation
   - ⚪ unacceptable documentation

> **Standard 8**: All entries in the medical record should be permanent.

3. The hospital administrator was informed by the health information manager that several physicians were altering patients' medical records incorrectly. The hospital administrator drafted a policy to these physicians stating that all entries in the medical record are permanent. Following the implementation of this policy the physicians stopped altering the medical records incorrectly.
   - ⚪ acceptable documentation
   - ⚪ unacceptable documentation

> **Standard 7**: Only abbreviations and symbols approved by the organization and/or medical staff rules and regulations should be used in the medical record.

4. While John was coding a medical record he noticed several abbreviations with which he was not familiar. He looked these up to see if they were approved by the hospital and they were, so he did not expand them in the patient's medical record.
   - ⚪ acceptable documentation
   - ⚪ unacceptable documentation

> **Standard 3**: Only individuals authorized by the organization's policies should be allowed to enter documentation in the medical record.

5. Susan performed an audit of several medical records to determine if the individuals who made entries in these medical records were authorized by the hospital to enter documentation in these records. She compared the list of authorized individuals with those who documented information in these records and determined that several of the individuals were not on the approved list.
    - ○ acceptable documentation
    - ○ unacceptable documentation

Documentation Consistency and Auditing

Let's look at a couple more points on the general documentation standards. The first relates to the first standard, "…the uniformity of both the content and the format of the medical record." In health information management, "uniformity of content" does not mean every patient has to get sick with the same thing! **Uniformity of content** or **vocabulary standards** means that common definitions of medical terms that encourage consistent descriptions of a patient's condition in the medical record are used. Still clear as mud? What does that mean? In simple terms, it means healthcare documentation should use the common and acceptable medical terms for describing patient conditions and treatments.

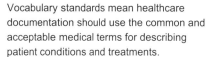

Highlights

Vocabulary standards mean healthcare documentation should use the common and acceptable medical terms for describing patient conditions and treatments.

Slang terms, ambiguous, uncommon, or unusual terms should be avoided, and consistent, clear language should be used within a report to describe a patient's condition and treatment. As a transcriptionist, your knowledge of anatomy, pathophysiology, pharmacology, and medical language will be invaluable in assuring your knowledge of the vocabulary standards.

The second of the "couple more points" relates to standard #11, "… develop, implement, and evaluate policies and procedures related to the qualitative and quantitative analysis of medical records." This is a check, check, and double check principle. Medical records should be reviewed while they are being created, while they are being compiled, and after their completion. Medical records documentation audits of individual records and provider records should be done consistently.

On the previous page, we had a highlight box with definitions of *qualitative analysis* and *quantitative analysis*. Go back and review them and see if you can figure out which definition goes with which word below.

Challenge Box

1. DEFINITION 1: Review of the medical record to ensure that standards are met and to determine accuracy of record documentation.
2. DEFINITION 2: Review of the medical record to determine its completeness.

How did you do? I am sure that your knowledge of vocabulary helped out. Qualitative deals with the *quality* of the information in the record. Quanitative deals with the *quantity* of information in the record.

There are three other types of reviews or audits you should be aware of:

Review or Audit	Meaning
Concurrent review	Review of the medical record carried out while the patient is actively receiving care.
Occurrence screening	Review technique of medical records of current and discharged patients with the goal of identifying events which could potentially lead to compensation by the healthcare provider.
Retrospective review	Review of the medical record after the patient has been discharged.

Concurrent reviews are conducted while the patient is receiving treatment. HIM professionals and document authors review the records as they are created and compiled. The benefit of this type of review is that documentation issues can be identified at the time of patient care and rectified (if necessary) in a timely manner.

Occurrence screening is a **risk management-related** audit. The reviewer looks for accidents, omissions, or medical errors which resulted or could potentially result in a personal injury or loss of property. Occurrences include instances when the wrong surgery was performed or when an informed consent for a procedure was not obtained.

Retrospective review does not allow for timely identification of documentation issues, but it is still very useful for identifying and addressing weaknesses in documentation processes, areas where staff need additional training and, where appropriate, addressing deficiencies in individual records.

I. MATCHING.
Match the term and the definition. Enter the letter for the corresponding definition next to the term.

1. ____ concurrent review
2. ____ documentation standards
3. ____ acceptable documentation
4. ____ qualitative analysis
5. ____ The Joint Commission
6. ____ occurrence screening
7. ____ unacceptable documentation
8. ____ retrospective review
9. ____ vocabulary standards
10. ____ quantitative analysis

A. Complete, legible, and chronological account of patient care.
B. Incomplete or unclear information in a medical record.
C. Organization which accredits hospitals based on accreditation standards.
D. Medical record review performed after the patient has been discharged.
E. Review of the medical record to identify potential medical errors.
F. Common definitions of medical terms in the patient's medical record.
G. Review of the medical record while the patient is still a patient.
H. Developed to ensure the uniformity, accuracy, and completeness of medical record entries.
I. Review of medical record to ensure that documentation standards are met.
J. Medical record review for completeness.

Risk Management

Adherence to documentation standards creates an environment for quality patient care. Organizations and healthcare providers adopt and maintain rigorous documentation standards for other important reasons.

Think back to our examples at the beginning of the module. Do you remember the patient who had the wrong leg operated on? As you can imagine, this would not only ruin the patient's day, it would probably make for a long and frustrating day, week, month, and year for the healthcare provider. Quality, accurate healthcare documentation protects the patient, but it also protects the provider. The concept of applying medical, legal, and administrative operations within a healthcare organization to minimize the exposure to liability is known as **risk management**.

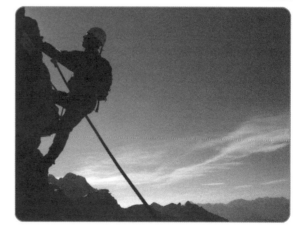

A good **risk management** program holds everyone—doctors, nurses, staff—accountable and reduces the risk of lawsuits and patient care errors.

Quality healthcare documentation practices minimize the potential for **fraud and abuse.** Individuals, state and local governments, as well as private insurance companies, spend billions of dollars annually for healthcare services. Excellent healthcare documentation means healthcare providers can support the medical bills with clear, accurate records and are more likely to receive full reimbursement for their services. Claims can be denied or payment reduced if complete, accurate documentation does not support the healthcare charges.

Highlights

The concept of applying medical, legal, and administrative operations within a healthcare organization to minimize the exposure to liability is known as **risk management**.

Government auditors and accrediting organizations look very closely at medical records to determine if the healthcare provider is changing, manipulating, or altering diagnosis or treatment records to receive inappropriate reimbursement. **Fraud and abuse** detection and prevention are benefits of a well-managed risk management program.

Documentation Errors

The job of implementing and managing the documentation standards will not usually be the job of the medical transcriptionist (although some medical transcriptionists choose the career path of HIM department manager or risk management supervisor). To be effective and efficient as a transcriptionist and ensure quality documentation, you need to become familiar with common documentation errors and deficiencies. The following is a list of these common errors and deficiencies:

- Missing/incorrect patient identification (name, medical record number, gender, etc.)
- Diagnoses/procedures or other text inconsistencies, ambiguities, or insufficiencies
- Missing physician signatures
- Location discrepancies (left/right, inconsistencies in description of wound or illness)
- Date inconsistencies

When these types of errors or deficiencies are identified in the patient's medical record, they need to be reported. (Of note, in the educational setting you will not have access to full patient medical records and confidential information.) Most healthcare organizations have developed automated systems for tracking errors or deficiencies. Health information personnel create a **deficiency slip** indicating the error or deficiency. This slip is placed in the patient's medical record, and the record is filed in a specially designated area of the HIM department. This is commonly known as the **incomplete record file.** The physician, the appropriate HIMs staff, or the appropriate healthcare provider accesses the incomplete record file to provide clarification, additional information, or whatever is necessary to correct or complete the file.

A tool often used by transcriptionists and medical coding specialists, is the **physician query** form. A physician query is used when the transcriptionist requires additional information or a clarification to appropriately transcribe the patient's medical record. In a small office, MTs often have the ability to simply ask the physician. In larger offices or a remote transcription setting, a form is used to request additional information from the physician.

The physician query becomes a permanent part of the medical record. When a physician responds to a physician query, the risk management supervisor typically uses the information to make any appropriate changes to the record.

Each employer will have a system for identifying and addressing medical record documentation issues, as well as a system for inquiring of the physician when more information is needed.

I. MULTIPLE CHOICE.
Review the following reports and answer the questions below.

Documentation – Scenario 1

Medical Record

Procedure Note

PATIENT NAME:

MEDICAL RECORD NUMBER: 18-65-76

OPERATION DATE: 8/25/2001

SURGEON: Dr. Smith

PREOPERATIVE DIAGNOSIS: Obstruction in esophagus due to carcinoma.

PROCEDURE PERFORMED: Dilatation of esophagus and replacement of nasogastric feeding tube.

FINDINGS: This patient had radiation therapy for squamous cell carcinoma located in the mid thorax beginning at below the aortic arch. The radiation therapy has not opened the esophagus and the patient cannot swallow satisfactorily around the 18-French nasogastric tube. The patient was brought in for dilation of his esophagus and possible pharyngogastric tube insertion; however, the patient developed tachycardia and shortness of breath and it appeared that his condition was fragile.

It is known this patient has severe coronary artery disease with ejection fraction of 15% and cardiomyopathy of severe degree. Therefore, the procedure was stopped after dilating the esophagus up to 30-French.

The nasogastric tube, which was previously placed and pulled back up, was passed down into the stomach and fixed in this position. The patient tolerated the procedure satisfactorily, although the full extent of the planned surgery was not performed. The patient's pulse returned back to 100 with no change in blood pressure with nasal oxygen saturation remaining normal. The patient was sent to post-anesthesia care unit.

1. What information is incorrect or missing from this report?

   ○ operation date
   ○ patient name
   ○ medical record number
   ○ preoperative diagnosis

Documentation – Scenario 2

Medical Record

Clinic Note

PATIENT NAME: John Smith

MEDICAL RECORD NUMBER: 25-85-96

DATE: 2/18/2004

PHYSICIAN: Dr. Jones

HISTORY: This is a 54-year-old male with a history of seizure disorder, likely etiology was alcohol related. No history of head injury or coma. She has not had any seizures in more than six months. He has slowed down on his alcohol use and is complaining of some dizziness, usually worsened with a quick change in position. She has also quit smoking and is using the patch. He was on Neurontin, but it has been discontinued. He is currently taking doxepin 150 mg h.s.

Neurological exam is unremarkable, and there is no change from the previous visit.

ASSESSMENT: Dizziness

PLAN: If EEG (electroencephalogram) is negative, plan to give Antivert 12.5 to 25 mg p.o. p.r.n. for dizziness. Again, I stressed to her to stop drinking. His follow up appointment will be in six months.

2. What information is incorrect or missing from this report?

   ○ patient name
   ○ date
   ○ gender inconsistency
   ○ medical record number

Technology and Patient Confidentiality

Now that we've talked about documentation standards, risk management, and the role of the medical transcriptionist in identifying and addressing common documentation errors, we're going to talk about another critically important issue and professional responsibility of the MT: assuring patient confidentiality.

At the beginning of this unit, we presented four scenarios to illustrate the importance of accuracy, timeliness, and confidentiality. The last two scenarios illustrate the unforeseen, but potentially devastating, consequences of compromised record security and patient confidentiality.

Scenario 3:

Kelly visits a local clinic for blood work and learns she has AIDS. The clinic's computer is "hacked " into and her personal information and AIDS status are printed on an anti-homosexual flyer in her hometown.

Scenario 4:

Your husband suffers from depression. He is treated with medication and counseling and copes well with family and work. He applies for a promotion but it is denied because his boss heard from his neighbor, a nurse who works where your husband receives his medical care, about his depression and thinks it might affect his ability to do a good job.

Every medical transcriptionist has a very serious responsibility to protect patient confidentiality. This responsibility is professional, legal, and ethical in nature. The MT must be aware of the responsibilities and potential consequences related to patient confidentiality. In recent years, political, professional, and technological changes have altered the landscape of patient records and the confidentiality of these records.

Not so very long ago, when information in patient medical records was all stored on paper and was only transferable to other healthcare providers via confidential mail and private telephone calls, it was relatively difficult for outsiders to gain access to it. Of course, this meant it wasn't particularly easy for those who needed access to information to get it either! Healthcare providers, like consulting physicians and nurses, had to wait for the piece of paperwork to be found and shuffled around to get the information they needed.

> ### Highlights
>
> Technology has enabled exciting breakthroughs for patients and the medical community, such as video conferencing. Video conferencing allows physicians an opportunity to consult "face-to-face" with their patients, other professionals, or both. In some cases, video conferencing has enabled "supervised" medical procedures to be performed in remote areas under the direction of capable clinicians, nurses, or physicians. This technology has been instrumental in saving lives.

Now information can be instantly transferred via e-mail, fax, Internet, voice files, video, and even small hand-held portable devices.

These miracles of modern technology have enhanced the opportunities for collaboration because patient information can be shared quickly for the best possible medical care available. It is really exciting to think about! You can be on vacation virtually anywhere in the world, and your provider can instantly access your records or otherwise exchange vital medical information about you with your hometown doctor. For those with complex medical histories or multiple medical problems, this can mean the difference between life and death.

However, there's a tradeoff to having easily available information and that tradeoff is **security**. The free flow of information means there is an increased risk of personal data and medical details being intercepted. Not a comfortable feeling, but there's no turning back—and we wouldn't want to. As long as the potential risks of electronically transferred data are managed, technology provides enhanced health information management and information sharing.

EHR and Its Benefits

The **EHR**, or **electronic health record**, is a medical record that exists entirely in electronic format. A patient's EHR can be a compilation of information from a single visit or contain information from multiple healthcare-related visits. Most healthcare providers are somewhere in-between an entirely paper-based system and a completely computer-based (electronic) system.

Medical record numbers are unique numbers used to identify individual recipients of healthcare services. If a national electronic health record system is adopted, each person would likely have a **universal personal identifier** which would uniquely identify him or her at ANY provider of healthcare services.

In the near future, more and more healthcare providers will migrate to electronic health records to store and transmit their patients' health information. Standard accepted practices, known as **health informatics standards**, for collecting, maintaining, and transferring healthcare information among computer systems make it possible for healthcare providers to select and maintain an appropriate EHR system for their documentation needs. It is critical to note that *there is currently no national standard electronic health record system.* There is public and industry-wide discussion, and a generally widely held belief, that a "universal" electronic health record will be adopted in the future.

There are many benefits for healthcare providers to switch from a **paper-based record** (medical record data printed and stored on paper in a hard copy format) to an **electronic-based record** (medical record data stored in an electronic format in a computer system or systems). These benefits include the following:

Ease of storage – The more visits a patient makes to his or her healthcare provider, the larger the patient's medical record becomes. Many healthcare providers see hundreds or even thousands of patients. Record storage can take up a lot of space in any office. Storing patients' health information in an electronic health record (EHR) simply saves space.

Accessibility – Authorized users can access EHR information from on-site or remote computers. If a healthcare provider needs information, they no longer have to physically go to a record storage area or request a file clerk retrieve documents from a physical record in a records room. Authorized users have immediate access to information. Information is stored and indexed for easy retrieval "on demand."

Efficiency – Easy access leads directly to efficiency. As soon as information is entered, it's accessible. The end user (patient, physician) does not have to wait for the document to travel from healthcare provider to medical transcriptionist to medical coder to medical biller before they have access to it. The original document is available and additions can be made efficiently until the document reaches a final form.

Searchability – It takes less time to search for a specific item in an electronic document than in a hard copy document. Software tools and features make searching quick and easy. This is a benefit for providing patient care to an individual patient and it is a time saver as well.

Uniformity and standardization – As mentioned previously, it is widely believed that adoption of a national electronic health record system will take place in a matter of time. In the meantime, most electronic health record systems adhere to **structure and content standards**—common elements and definitions to be included in an electronic health record. Many computer programs used for electronic record management control the fields to be entered, the order the information is to be entered, and the presentation of information on the screen. This way two doctors who would otherwise present their information in completely different formats will have uniform records.

Collaboration – Accessibility and efficiency make collaboration and information sharing easier. Many providers can simultaneously view a record simply by accessing the record electronically. This collaborative process—or the use of information technology to improve the quality, safety, efficiency, and confidentiality of healthcare through simultaneous access to patient health information by multiple healthcare providers—is known as **health information exchange**.

Reduction in medical errors – When records are available quickly, are easily searched, and are easily updated, the opportunities for patient care errors are reduced. Additionally, handwritten entries in a patient record can be challenging to read. (Have you ever tried to decipher a signature on your prescription slip?) A totally integrated EHR does away with handwritten entries and reduces the risk of errors made trying to decipher illegible scrawl.

I. MATCHING.
Match the correct term to the definition.

1. ___ health informatics standards
2. ___ electronic health record
3. ___ health information exchange
4. ___ paper-based record
5. ___ uniformity

A. Overall regularity that is found in many electronic health records.

B. Record of a patient's health information which is created and stored in a computer.

C. Medical record data printed and stored on paper.

D. Simultaneous access to a patient's health information to improve the quality of healthcare.

E. Standards developed to collect and transfer healthcare information between computer systems.

EHR Challenges

We don't want to talk about the roses and skip the thorns—so let's look at some of the challenges to be managed with electronic records. The technology driving the EHRs is developing and changing rapidly. As with any new product, there is always a period of trial when mistakes, shortcomings, and unforseen problems arise. Have you ever received one of those recall notices in the mail concerning an issue discovered with your automobile? With technology, the issues are slightly different than with automobiles. Programs and hardware must be able to keep accurate records that can be shared with the *right* people without falling victim to crashes, viruses, or hacking.

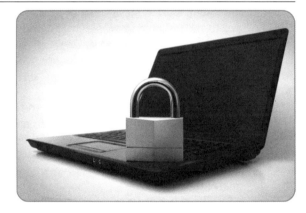

The major concerns with the EHR are as follows:

Cost – The main disadvantage to fully implementing an EHR is the cost. There is no national standardized EHR program (although this is an initiative being discussed at national, state, and local levels, as well as in industry groups, such as The Joint Commission). So designing, implementing, and maintaining an EHR is a significant undertaking. Healthcare providers must invest dollars to develop or purchase, then install and maintain an EHR system that adequately meets their needs.

Confidentiality and security – The biggest concerns are maintaining confidentiality and security of the patient's health information. Identity theft and unauthorized use of personal information are constantly in the news. In fact, in 2006, there was a well-publicized case of a worker in a Veterans' Administration hospital who took home the personal data and medical information on thousands of veterans.

Security of all types of information is important in today's world. With the rise of identity theft and insurance fraud, companies and individuals are constantly seeking ways to ensure information security. Unfortunately, as we often see in the news, security and confidentiality are not always maintained. You may remember the following bit of news.

Federal officials yesterday announced the recovery of computer equipment stolen from an employee of the Department of Veterans Affairs. They said that sensitive personal information of 26.5 million veterans and military personnel apparently had not been accessed.

The laptop and external hard drive, stolen May 3, [2006] from a VA data analyst's home in Aspen Hill, contained the names, birth dates and Social Security numbers of millions of current and former service members. The theft was the largest information security breach in government history and raised fears of potential mass identity theft.

VA Secretary Jim Nicholson announced the recovery yesterday during a hearing of the House Committee on Veterans Affairs. *

*("Stolen VA Laptop and Hard Drive Recovered." The Washington Post. http://www.washingtonpost.com/wp-dyn/content/article/2006/06/29/AR2006062900352.html)

Let's face it. It would have been much more difficult for this data analyst to take home 26.5 million hard copy records!

A series of privacy laws over the years has sought to address the issues of security and confidentiality—eventually leading to the drafting and implementation of the **Health Insurance Portability and Accountability Act (HIPAA)**, the law that protects confidentiality and security of electronically transmitted information. We will delve into HIPAA in greater detail next.

I. **MULTIPLE CHOICE.**
    Choose the best answer.

    1. Which of the following would not be considered a benefit when utilizing the electronic health record?
        ◯ It is easy to store information.
        ◯ It is easy to locate information.
        ◯ It is easy access for patient, family members, and friends.
        ◯ It is easy for others to read the medical record.

    2. The EHR makes it easier to _____.
        ◯ read the physician's orders
        ◯ get information about the patient from other healthcare facilities
        ◯ get the patient's medical record quickly
        ◯ all of the above

3. HIPAA is _____.

   ○ a computer program used to ensure uniformity of medical records
   ○ a law protecting confidentiality of patient records
   ○ a government oversight agency charged with changing paper records to electronic records
   ○ an acronym used to identify a security breach

4. A prime concern related to an electronic health record is _____.

   ○ speed and accessibility
   ○ the inability to share information
   ○ security and confidentiality
   ○ computer capabilities

5. Which would NOT be considered a problem associated with implementation of the EHR?

   ○ The cost of designing, implementing and maintaining the electronic record.
   ○ Maintaining confidentiality.
   ○ Finding a place to store the electronic records.
   ○ Controlling access to the electronic record.

HIPAA

Now that you have some background information, we can move on to HIPAA, patient privacy, and confidentiality.

The federal government has enacted a series of laws designed to protect an individual's privacy. These include The Privacy Act of 1974, The Privacy Act of 1993, and the **Health Insurance Portability and Accountability Act** of 1996, which is generally known as **HIPAA**.

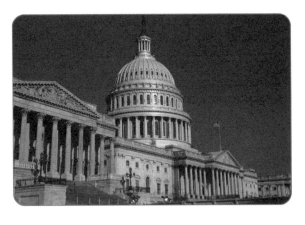

You are probably familiar with the Fourth Amendment. It guarantees "the right of the people to be secure in their persons, houses, papers and effects…" In other words, the Constitution specifically protects all of us from information about our private lives being made available in the public domain. The Privacy Acts of 1974 and 1993 are general laws designed to protect an individual's right to keep these private matters—private. These include information related to one's employment, religion, or medical history. You are probably aware, through television and movies if not directly from your physician, that doctors are "not allowed" to give any detail of your medical problems or history to anyone not involved in your care or not authorized by you. For many years the healthcare industry operated with a fairly clear understanding of the nature and extent of these laws, as well as any penalty which may result from a failure to comply with them.

In 1996, the federal government decided that the existing laws were insufficient to deal with the reality of the threat technology poses to privacy, and specifically to the privacy of a patient's health record. The government believes that not having a guarantee of privacy has a detrimental effect on receiving effective medical care. Basically, if you are afraid that your health information is going to be made public, you may not tell your physician what is really wrong, may not have tests that are important to your care and treatment, or may not even go to a practitioner at all.

There has been quite a bit of press coverage (especially in the medical coding and medical transcription industries) about the resultant legislation—HIPAA (This is pronounced as one word "hippa"). Although it was passed in 1996, the time frame for healthcare organizations, insurance companies, facilities, and practitioners to become compliant was April 14, 2003.

There are three main goals that HIPAA is to achieve:

Goals of HIPAA

1. Give people access to their own health information and control others' access.

2. Enable patients to trust the healthcare system to keep their medical records confidential.

3. Make healthcare better and more efficient by putting privacy protection into a national framework.

There are four major reasons provided in the Privacy Rule as to why the government believes that these changes are necessary. These include:

Reasons for HIPAA

1. More organizations are involved in the provision of care and the processing of claims.

2. The growing use of electronic information technology.

3. Increased efforts to market healthcare (and other products) to consumers.

4. Increased availability of highly sensitive medical information due to advances in scientific research.

In many ways technology has dramatically improved healthcare. As we discussed earlier, however, there are inadvertent and often unintentional side effects of the availability of information. For example, as technology improves and businesses, healthcare facilities, and individuals upgrade their equipment, old computers often contain the private information that was stored on them. It is possible that a doctor could sell (or even give away) an old computer without realizing that confidential records are still accessible. There is also more sinister and deliberate mismanagement of patient information. Some specific examples of clear breaches to privacy which contributed to the need for HIPAA are cited in the Privacy Rule. Here are a few of them:

- The *Ann Arbor News* reported in February 1999 that a Michigan-based health system accidentally posted the medical records of thousands of patients on the Internet.
- The *New York Times* reported in August 1991 that a speculator bid $4,000 for the patient records of a family practice in South Carolina. Among the businessman's uses of the purchased records was to sell them back to the former patients.
- The *National Law Journal*, May 30, 1994, cited a banker who also sat on a county health board gained access to patients' records and identified several people with cancer and called in their mortgages.

Frightening, isn't it? HIPAA, at least ideally, should curtail some of these privacy breaches. It provides penalties—both civil and criminal—for the misuse of private medical information. Civil penalties can be incurred of not more than $100 per violation, totaling not more than $25,000 per year. Criminal penalties are much stiffer. A basic violation can include a fine of up to $50,000 and/or up to a year in prison. Using health information under false pretenses can carry penalties of up to $100,000 and/or 5 years in prison. Violations involving the use of private health information for commercial gain or malicious harm can carry fines of up to $250,000 and/or 10 years in prison. In other words, the rule has some teeth.

I. **TRUE/FALSE.**
Mark the following true or false.

1. HIPAA was enacted by the federal government.
   ○ true
   ○ false

2. A goal of HIPAA is to make healthcare better and more efficient.
   ○ true
   ○ false

3. HIPAA regulations are enforced by law, but there are no penalties for infractions of the law.
   ○ true
   ○ false

4. Increased use of technology in the medical record is one of the reasons HIPAA was enacted.
   ○ true
   ○ false

5. You need to know about HIPAA because your healthcare provider is not responsible for informing you of your privacy rights.
   ○ true
   ○ false

Internal Facility Policies

The HIPAA Privacy Rule requires that all facilities, businesses, and individuals who have access to health records abide by the rule (obviously). As a medical transcriptionist, you fall under this category. Whether you work for a clinic, a hospital, a private transcription company, or for yourself, the company for whom you work will have created a series of policies and procedures that will put them into compliance with HIPAA regulations. They **should** make you aware of these policies, but if they do not, **you must** know your responsibilities regarding patient and medical record privacy. Asking your employer about their privacy policies is a good first step. Knowing the law and being vigilant about confidentiality is the next step.

If you work in a facility, you should be trained by the facility; however, as a conscientious person, you would ask to be trained on their privacy policies if the training is not provided as part of your orientation. If you work from home, you should be given explicit instructions from the service or clinic that hires you; again, if they don't, it is still your responsibility to be compliant. There are some important guidelines that work-from-home transcriptionists must follow in their efforts to remain HIPAA compliant.

Discretion – Do not share any demographic, confidential, or otherwise revealing information, be it online (such as in forums), in e-mails, or verbally. This is strictly against HIPAA regulations and could result in penalties.

Access control – Do not allow anyone access to your computer. Your work computer holds medical reports containing sensitive, confidential information. This might mean you have a computer exclusively for work (in fact, some companies require you to have a computer that is used only for work).

Use of the Internet – There will be predetermined policies and procedures for connection to the Internet (for any reason) from a computer containing confidential patient information. This would allow protection of that information from viruses or hackers attempting to gain access to any computer connected to the Internet. Proper encryption is required to ensure information is secure during transfer.

Workplace security – Always use headphones when transcribing. If you can hear the report through your computer speakers, other people likely can hear it as well—yes, even the neighbor in the upstairs apartment! Your computer monitor should be placed in a private place where foot traffic will not be able to see the information on the screen. If you need to take a break from your work and leave the room, you should not leave your computer on. In your absence people would have access to your work.

As you can see, there are many possible ways that HIPAA may affect your job as an MT. The good news is that as an MT you will have access to HIPAA and its requirements. Your job will be to meet these requirements. Remember, not only are you protecting yourself, but all of the patients and healthcare services you are working for and with.

Patient Confidentiality

You already know HIPAA is a Privacy Rule enacted by the federal government to protect patient privacy. If you have received any healthcare services in the last few years, you should be somewhat familiar with HIPAA notices and policies. These are an effort by healthcare providers to comply with HIPAA standards. In fact, if patients are afraid their health problems will impact either their jobs or their position in the community, they will be much less likely to give accurate answers to questions asked by their practitioner regarding any health problem, and they may entirely avoid seeking professional help for it.

Okay, that makes sense. Patients should be able to trust their doctors to keep confidences. Most people are aware a physician, nurse, or other type of practitioner is required to keep their patient information **strictly** confidential. But how does that extend to you as a medical transcriptionist constantly working with patient records?

First and foremost, you will have to be familiar with and abide by the policies and procedures of your facility. You should also be required to sign a confidentiality form stating that you understand records are confidential and that you will abide by the policies and procedures of the facility/employer. Employers generally go about this in one of two ways:

1. You sign and date an actual copy of the policy statement with all details spelled out on the part of the form you affix your signature to.
2. You receive a separate copy of the policies and procedures of your employer and sign an acknowledgment that you did receive it and you read it.

Although the policy statements for every place you work will differ, the individual components should be largely the same. It will be important for you to understand what the individual issues are, the terminology associated with confidentiality, and the applicability to your position.

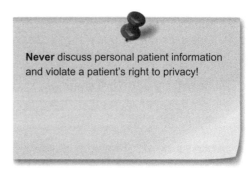

Never discuss personal patient information and violate a patient's right to privacy!

Let's assume you work with patient records every day. Confidential patient records. You see their names, their medical histories, their current problems, and their family histories—in other words, all manner of private information.

Some of the records you read will be interesting. Very interesting. Interesting to the point that you will want to talk to others about them. This is really good dish! You've got to hear this! *Avoid the temptation.* If you do speak to anyone outside of the healthcare professionals who are also managing the patient's care about information contained in a medical record, you must *never* discuss it using the names or *any other identifying details* of the patient.

You have to be careful because it is possible to make clear who a patient is without ever saying the patient's name or age. For example, you could say, "A middle-aged white male from Texas whose father was also President of the United States…" No names. No dates. No age. Who is being discussed?

It's a small world—the friend you speak with might be the brother of a cousin's friend of a former spouse's sister—you can't know. It's important to be absolutely exact in maintaining patient confidentiality.

I. MULTIPLE CHOICE.
Choose the best answer.

1. Privacy is _____.
   ○ a fundamental right
   ○ covered in the 4th amendment
   ○ to be protected
   ○ all of the above

2. When was HIPAA implemented?
   ○ in 1974
   ○ in 1993
   ○ in 2003
   ○ in 1996

3. Within the Privacy Rules, which is not a justification for HIPAA?
   ○ Protect consumer rights by providing access to their medical records.
   ○ Control the inappropriate use of that information.
   ○ Restore trust in the government.
   ○ Create a national framework for health privacy protection.

4. Which is not considered a reason for implementation of HIPAA rules?

   ○ Advances in scientific research and increased use of electronic technology.
   ○ Increased desire to market healthcare products to the consumer.
   ○ More insurance companies handling medical claims.
   ○ Restrict healthcare provider's ability to file medical claims.

5. Preventing breach of privacy is one of the primary goals of the Privacy Rule. Which would be considered a breach of privacy?

   ○ Sharing medical information between physicians.
   ○ Asking a physician for clarity on a medical report.
   ○ Leaving your work computer on when you take a break.
   ○ Typing a dictated medical report.

6. Working as a transcriptionist requires knowledge about policies and procedures of your employer. These would include _____.

   ○ access control
   ○ transfer of data
   ○ use of the Internet
   ○ all of the above

7. Which would not be considered a violation of confidentiality?

   ○ Providing your sign-on code and password to a friend.
   ○ Using another person's sign-on code and password.
   ○ Asking a friend about a patient and his illness.
   ○ Asking the physician to clarify an unclear word in a report.

8. Violating Privacy Rules can result in _____.

   ○ loss of your job
   ○ a major fine
   ○ going to jail
   ○ all of the above

9. A Statement of Policy usually includes which of the following?

   ○ A formal job description for a transcriptionist.
   ○ Your financial remuneration as a transcriptionist.
   ○ Penalties for breach of the policy.
   ○ The responsibility of employees.

10. An acknowledgment of responsibility is _____.

    ○ a statement of the employee's legal and ethical guidelines
    ○ a form provided to the patient to be signed
    ○ a list of what treatment the patient will receive
    ○ a list of the rules to be followed at the facility

Patient Information and Interaction

Okay—after the serious nature of our discussion, it seems to be time for a laugh.

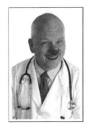

Medical Humor

"A patient in New York went to a doctor for a checkup. The doctor wrote out a prescription for him in his usual illegible handwriting. The man put it in his pocket and forgot to have it filled. Every morning for two years he showed it to the conductor as a railroad pass. Twice it got him into the Radio City Music Hall, once into a baseball park, and once into a symphony concert. One day he mislaid it at home, and his daughter picked it up, played it on the piano, and won a scholarship to a music conservatory."

Ah, medical humor. You have to love it. Let's get back to work.

There are times that patients need to give their medical information to someone else—perhaps another medical facility or an individual. Since this information is highly sensitive, there are guidelines that need to be followed when releasing medical information. There are two primary ways in which consent can be given by the patient for medical and personal information to be released: written consent and implied consent.

Written consent is when a patient signs a **release of information (ROI)** form authorizing his/her healthcare provider to release or send medical information to a particular individual or another healthcare provider for a specific purpose. These forms are most commonly used: 1) when patients need to have their information sent to a new healthcare provider (most often encountered when changing providers); 2) when patients are referred to a specialist for additional or consulting care that cannot be provided by their general practitioner; 3) when a lawsuit is in process and access to vital medical information is needed by attorneys; 4) to allow the healthcare provider to submit medical claims to insurance companies for reimbursement and to answer any questions they may have regarding the patient's medical care, diagnoses, or prognosis. Of course, there are other reasons written consent may be needed in order to transfer a patient's confidential medical information.

Implied consent is when a patient consents to disclosure of confidential medical information without signing an official release of information form. This type of consent usually occurs when patients are seen and treated in medical settings that require those who assist with their care to be informed of their conditions and treatment plans (e.g. assisting physicians, surgeons, nurses, and technicians). Consent is also implied when patients are transferred from one healthcare provider or medical facility to another and the new provider or medical facility must have access to the patient's medical information in order to ensure continuation of care.

There are times a provider may legally disclose confidential patient information without either written or implied consent and not get into trouble. These situations are both legally and ethically justifiable due to overriding social considerations or concerns. These are normally safety issues, such as patients who are threatening serious bodily harm or injury to others or to themselves. In these instances, the attending physician or healthcare professional is justified in notifying the proper authorities and/or even the intended victim(s) of such a possibility. Additionally, patients who have contracted communicable diseases are also to be reported immediately to the Center for Disease Control so proper disease controls can be implemented to keep the disease from spreading and infecting many individuals. There are some instances in which social concerns outweigh patient privacy and confidentiality issues.

As a medical transcriptionist, you will be acting on behalf of patients and will be hearing and seeing information about those patients that is considered private and personal. Such information, if not kept confidential, can cause problems not only for the patient, but for the provider as well. In terms of patient confidentiality, we tend to think in terms of the big-ticket items: this person has AIDS, cancer, or suicidal tendencies. However, there are several ways issues of patient confidentiality intersect in a medical office or

150

facility, and they are all equally important in terms of confidentiality. Information pertaining to appointments, finances, insurance information, family relationships, addresses, phone numbers, and even basic treatment plans all fall under the scope of protected private information.

I. **MATCHING.**
   Match the correct term to the definition.

1. ___ confidential

2. ___ release of information

3. ___ employee confidentiality agreement

4. ___ authorization

5. ___ written consent

6. ___ security

7. ___ implied consent

A. form employees sign that contracts them to comply with the rules, regulations, and laws surrounding patient privacy standards

B. unwritten patient consent that allows individuals involved in the patient's care and treatment access to personal medical information

C. permission by the patient to use or disclose his/her health information

D. privileged patient information

E. protection of data, information, and information networks from unauthorized use

F. a form with patient signature consenting for personal patient information to be released to a specified facility or individual

G. written patient permission to copy medical information

Professional MT Ethics

Since this unit is called Medical Ethics and Confidentiality, you can't be finished with the unit until you've considered ethics! Ethics has little to do with memorizing laws about patient or employer rights and a great deal to do with an individual's personal commitment to having integrity in his/her professional conduct. Let's begin by defining two important terms:

Ethics – a principle of right or good conduct.

Professional ethics – the principles and standards that underlie one's responsibilities and conduct in a particular field of expertise (profession).

Professional ethics is about setting a personal standard to abide by when asked to apply laws, rules, or guidelines and a personal standard to abide by in the absence of laws, rules, or guidelines.

As a transcriptionist, you will hear and have access to highly sensitive medical information about individuals. You are required by law not to discuss the nature of anyone's chart with any other person, including the individual whose chart it is. Medical transcriptionists are guardians of patient rights, both moral and legal, and ethical medical transcriptionists protect patient privacy, work with care providers to fortify patient safety, public health, and quality care.

As a working MT you will undoubtedly have ethical standards set by the company or facility you are transcribing for. AHDI (Association for Healthcare Documentation Integrity) has also published a standards of conduct and ethical principles for the medical transcriptionist professional.

I. TRUE/FALSE.
Mark the following true or false.

1. All MTs follow one set code of ethics.

    ○ true
    ○ false

2. It is okay to discuss a patient's medical chart with the patient.

    ○ true
    ○ false

3. Ethics, in general, involve good conduct.

    ○ true
    ○ false

4. You will not be exposed to personal or confidential information as an MT.

    ○ true
    ○ false

5. Ethics have to do with an individual's commitment to integrity and professional conduct.

    ○ true
    ○ false

152

II. MULTIPLE CHOICE.
Using the AHDI Code of Ethics, choose the best answer.

1. It is important to respect the rights and (◯dignity, ◯desires) of all individuals.

2. One should strive to provide accurate and (◯timeless, ◯timely) information.

3. One should (◯endorse, ◯implement) and maintain standards of professional transcription practice.

4. It is important to exercise (◯integrity, ◯interest) in all professional practices.

5. One should (◯comply with, ◯document) laws, regulations, and standards of patient documentation.

Answer Key

Work Types – Introduction

I. TRUE/FALSE.
1. false
2. false
3. true
4. false
5. false
6. true
7. false
8. false
9. true
10. true

Report Components

Clinic Note Components

I. MULTIPLE CHOICE.
1. How the physician interprets the findings; an opinion, impression, assessment, or diagnosis
2. Treatment and followup, including medication regimen, instruction, suggested education, and followup instruction
3. A narrative of the patient's own description of his/her compaints: a past history, review of systems, allergies, or medication lists
4. The description of the physician's findings on observation and examination, any physical signs, and laboratory testing or diagnostic studies, such as x-rays

Standard Acute Care Components

I. FILL IN THE BLANK.
1. History
2. Social History
3. Hospital course
4. Review of Systems
5. Chief Complaint
6. Physical Examination
7. Past Medical History
8. Medications
9. Plan
10. Surgical History
11. Diagnosis/Assessment
12. Family History
13. Diagnostic Studies
14. Allergies

Operative Note Components

I. MATCHING.
1. B. Preoperative Diagnosis
2. G. Postoperative Diagnosis
3. D. Operations
4. E. Surgeon
5. F. Assistant Surgeon(s)
6. I. Anesthesia
7. H. Estimated Blood Loss
8. C. Indication for Operation
9. J. Procedure
10. A. Findings

PE Abbreviations – Lesson 1

II. FILL IN THE BLANK.

1. clubbing, cyanosis, or edema
2. Bartholin glands, urethra, and Skene glands
3. tympanic membranes
4. auscultation and percussion
5. serous otitis media
6. regular rate and rhythm
7. blood pressure
8. arteriovenous
9. central nervous system
10. costovertebral angle

PE Abbreviations – Lesson 2

II. MATCHING.

1. A. HEENT
2. B. Neck
3. A. HEENT
4. D. Neurological
5. A. HEENT

PE Abbreviations – Lesson 3

II. FILL IN THE BLANK.

1. heart
2. normocephalic
3. joint
4. right
5. distress
6. delirium
7. eyes
8. jugular
9. left
10. ventricular

PE Abbreviations – Lesson 4

II. FILL IN THE BLANK.

1. right
2. breath
3. round
4. amputation
5. range
6. rapid
7. maximal
8. above
9. upper
10. lower

Physical Examination Samples

I. MULTIPLE CHOICE.

1. HEENT
2. head, eyes, ears, nose, throat
3. clubbing, cyanosis, or edema
4. genitourinary
5. PERRLA
6. RRR- regular rate and rhythm

Physical Examination Subheadings

I. TRUE/FALSE.

1. true
2. true
3. false
4. false

General and Vital Signs

I. MULTIPLE CHOICE.

1. hypotensive
2. cyanotic
3. state of alertness, personal hygiene, appearance, mood, etc.
4. Patient is 5 feet 6 inches, 175 pounds. Her blood pressure is 124/75.

HEENT

I. FILL IN THE BLANK.

1. Head
2. Nose
3. Eyes
4. Ears
5. Throat

Cardiovascular, Abdomen, and GU

I. MULTIPLE CHOICE.

1. fluid wave
2. heaves
3. perineal
4. Abdomen
5. Cardiovascular/Heart

Musculoskeletal

I. MULTIPLE CHOICE.

1. below-knee amputation
2. muscles, bones, and joints of the body
3. Palpation of the back reveals normal paraspinous muscle group with slight tenderness over C4.

Neurologic and Psychiatric

I. FILL IN THE BLANK.

1. nystagmus
2. tangential
3. neurologic
4. psychiatric

Review: Physical Examination Subheadings

I. SPELLING.

1. trachea midline
2. nontender
3. guaiac
4. clonus
5. carotid bruits
6. asymmetric
7. Romberg
8. posterior tibial
9. plantar
10. homicidal ideation

II. MULTIPLE CHOICE.

1. General
2. Neck
3. age
4. Musculoskeletal
5. eyes
6. Cardiovascular
7. Neck
8. HEENT
9. percussion
10. afebrile

Laboratory Data

Laboratory Abbreviations – Lesson 1

II. FILL IN THE BLANK.
1. dioxide
2. urea
3. count
4. arterial
5. sensitivity
6. bacillus

III. MULTIPLE CHOICE.
1. carbon
2. culture
3. arterial
4. count
5. urea

Laboratory Abbreviations – Lesson 2

II. FILL IN THE BLANK.
1. function
2. hemoglobin
3. immunodeficiency
4. cerebrospinal

III. MULTIPLE CHOICE.
1. hemoglobin
2. cerebrospinal
3. immunodeficiency
4. liver

Laboratory Abbreviations – Lesson 3

II. FILL IN THE BLANK.
1. prothrombin
2. thromboplastin
3. lumbar
4. ova
5. function
6. antigen

III. MULTIPLE CHOICE.
1. ova
2. function
3. partial
4. time
5. antigen

Laboratory Abbreviations – Lesson 4

II. FILL IN THE BLANK.
1. blood
2. tuberculosis
3. cells
4. urinalysis

III. MULTIPLE CHOICE.
1. urinalysis
2. red
3. white
4. tuberculosis

Basic Laboratory Studies – Lesson 1

I. MULTIPLE CHOICE.

1. hemoglobin and platelets
2. Beta HCG
3. ABG
4. Cardiac Studies
5. the time it takes for blood to clot
6. CMP
7. LP (lumbar puncture)
8. sodium, potassium, BUN, glucose, and calcium

Basic Laboratory Studies – Lesson 2

I. MULTIPLE CHOICE.

1. Endocrine
2. PSA
3. SMA
4. electrolytes
5. Lipid profile
6. Renal function tests
7. BUN
8. TIBC, ferritin, and transferrin
9. Urinalysis
10. LYTES
11. Hepatic function tests

Review: Laboratory Studies

I. MULTIPLE CHOICE.

1. sodium
2. TIBC
3. CBC
4. coagulation
5. drugs
6. overactive
7. SGOT/SGPT
8. blood urea nitrogen

II. TRUE/FALSE.

1. false
2. true
3. false
4. true

Lab Reports – Lesson 1

I. SPELLING.

1. sodium
2. bicarbonate
3. protein
4. hemoglobin
5. hematocrit
6. potassium
7. specific gravity
8. urinalysis
9. BUN
10. platelets

Lab Reports – Lesson 2

I. MULTIPLE CHOICE.

1. corpuscular
2. dioxide
3. urea
4. prothrombin
5. thromboplastin

Lab Reports – Lesson 3

I. MATCHING.

1. C. occult
2. F. glucose
3. G. electrolyte
4. A. atelectasis
5. E. creatinine
6. B. macrocytosis
7. D. platelets
8. H. white blood cells

Review: Normal Laboratory Values

I. MULTIPLE CHOICE.
1. hemoglobin
2. creatinine
3. hemoglobin 13
4. 37.2
5. hyperglycemic

II. TRUE/FALSE.
1. false
2. true
3. true
4. false
5. true

Formatting Guidelines

General Formatting Rules

I. TRUE/FALSE.
1. false
2. true
3. false
4. false
5. true

Review: Acronyms, Initialisms, Abbreviations, and Brief Forms

I. MULTIPLE CHOICE.
1. CABG
2. by mouth
3. A grouping of initials that you would NOT say aloud as you would an acronym.
4. brief form
5. b.i.d.

II. MATCHING.
1. C. n.r.
2. B. u.d.
3. E. p.c.
4. A. q.h.
5. D. gtt.

Review: Eponyms and Slang

I. MULTIPLE CHOICE.
1. micrograms
2. perf
3. Alzheimer
4. potassium chloride
5. differential
6. bundle of His
7. appy
8. dipyridamole sestamibi
9. eponym
10. sat

Review: Dangerous Abbreviations and Numbers

I. TRUE/FALSE.
1. false
2. true
3. false
4. false
5. true

1. hydrochlorothiazide
2. From 10% to 20%
3. The medication is to be taken 6 PM nightly
4. The patient was born in the 60s
5. She was given 10 mg of saline

Review: Lab Values and Headings

I. TRANSCRIPTION.
1. The hemoglobin and hematocrit were 12 and 36, respectively.
2. CARDIOVASCULAR: Regular rate and rhythm.
3. Specific gravity was 1.018.
4. His lab results revealed a pH of 7.1 and protein of 7 mg/dL.
5. HEENT

Review: Contractions, Hyphens, Genus, and Species

I. TRUE/FALSE.
1. false
2. true
3. true
4. false
5. true
6. false
7. false
8. true
9. false
10. true

Using Resources Effectively

Using Your Medical Dictionary

I. MULTIPLE CHOICE.
1. noun
2. relaxation
3. vomiting
4. cirrhoses
5. orange-yellow
6. liver
7. Latin OR Greek
8. crescent
9. knee
10. air
11. head
12. Arabic
13. foreign material in the GI tract
14. Ghana
15. a deficiency of calories and protein
16. retarded growth
17. matrices
18. tissue from which a structure develops
19. GI
20. gastrectomy
21. noun
22. glomeruli
23. kidney

There's A Medical Word For It

I. MATCHING.
1. V. pimple
2. N. baldness
3. P. headache
4. W. heel
5. B. heat
6. G. swallowing
7. I. nosebleed
8. S. belching
9. O. cross-eyed
10. Q. arm or leg

11.	M. stye	12.	T. dry, scaly skin
13.	U. freckles	14.	R. tongue
15.	D. urination	16.	Y. nostrils
17.	E. belly button	18.	X. eyelid
19.	F. fingers and toes	20.	J. sneezing
21.	H. redness	22.	K. athlete's foot
23.	C. hairball	24.	L. swelling
25.	A. wart		

Review: Google

I. TRUE/FALSE.

1. false
2. true
3. true
4. false
5. false

II. MATCHING.

1. D. Preferences
2. E. Minus sign
3. B. Answers.com
4. F. Advanced search
5. A. Plus sign
6. C. Google.com

Resource Challenge

I. MATCHING.

1. D. collyrium
2. A. Christmas disease
3. E. Einthoven's triangle
4. B. bovarism
5. F. subarachnoid cistern
6. C. fetal warfarin syndrome

Enunciation

I. TRUE/FALSE.

1. true
2. false
3. true
4. true
5. true

Phonetics (Fuh-net-icks)

I. FILL IN THE BLANK.

1. phosphatase
2. cerumen
3. adjuvant
4. Colles' OR Colles
5. rheumatic
6. Psoriasis
7. polydactyly
8. Pfannenstiel
9. xiphoid
10. chiasm
11. Vicryl
12. cecostomy
13. nabothian
14. graafian
15. Roux-en-Y
16. Klippel-Feil
17. moiety
18. fascicular
19. laryngeal
20. Schmorl's
21. Dupuytren's
22. Crohn's
23. Jackson-Pratt
24. carinatum
25. facetectomy
26. oscillating
27. papyracea
28. DeBakey
29. noxious
30. ecchymosis

31. Kaposi's	32. tinnitus
33. pterygium	34. scaphoid
35. aeruginosa	36. patulous
37. pes planum	38. Osgood-Schlatter's
39. emphysema	40. schwannoma
41. Vaccinations	42. Tinel's
43. Schatzki's	44. seborrheic
45. auricular	46. symphysis
47. dysgnathia	48. bougie
49. parenchymal	50. jaundice

Review: How to Look up Words

I. TRUE/FALSE.

1. false	2. true
3. true	4. false
5. false	

II. FILL IN THE BLANK.

1. Phalen	2. gestation
3. rales	4. Colles OR Colles'
5. amylase	6. hypertrophy
7. dorsiflexion	8. Doppler

Medical Ethics and Confidentiality

Documentation Standards

I. MULTIPLE CHOICE.

1. unacceptable documentation	2. unacceptable documentation
3. acceptable documentation	4. acceptable documentation
5. unacceptable documentation	

Documentation Consistency and Auditing

CHALLENGE BOX.

1. **Qualitative analysis** is the review of the medical record which deals with accuracy. Is the information contained correct and are the standards met?
2. **Quantitative analysis** is the review which deals with quantity or completeness of the record. Is everything there that should be?

I. MATCHING.

1. G. Review of the medical record while the patient is still a patient.

3. A. Complete, legible, and chronological account of patient care.
5. C. Organization which accredits hospitals based on accreditation standards.
7. B. Incomplete or unclear information in a medical record.
9. F. Common definitions of medical terms in the patient's medical record.

2. H. Developed to ensure the uniformity, accuracy, and completeness of medical record entries.
4. I. Review of medical record to ensure that documentation standards are met.
6. E. Review of the medical record to identify potential medical errors.
8. D. Medical record review performed after the patient has been discharged.
10. J. Medical record review for completeness.

Documentation Errors

I. MULTIPLE CHOICE.
1. patient name
2. gender inconsistency

Technology and Patient Confidentiality

I. TRUE/FALSE.
1. false
3. true
5. false
2. true
4. false

EHR and Its Benefits

I. MATCHING.
1. E. Standards developed to collect and transfer healthcare information between computer systems.
3. D. Simultaneous access to a patient's health information to improve the quality of healthcare.
5. A. Overall regularity that is found in many electronic health records.

2. B. Record of a patient's health information which is created and stored in a computer.
4. C. Medical record data printed and stored on paper.

EHR Challenges

I. MULTIPLE CHOICE.
1. It is easy access for patient, family members, and friends.
3. a law protecting confidentiality of patient records
5. Finding a place to store the electronic records.

2. all of the above
4. security and confidentiality

HIPAA

I. TRUE/FALSE.
1. true
3. false
5. false
2. true
4. true

Patient Confidentiality

I. MULTIPLE CHOICE.

1. all of the above
2. in 2003
3. Restore trust in the government.
4. Restrict healthcare provider's ability to file medical claims.
5. Leaving your work computer on when you take a break.
6. all of the above
7. Asking the physician to clarify an unclear word in a report.
8. all of the above
9. The responsibility of employees.
10. a statement of the employee's legal and ethical guidelines

Patient Information and Interaction

I. MATCHING.

1. D. privileged patient information
2. F. a form with patient signature consenting for personal patient information to be released to a specified facility or individual
3. A. form employees sign that contracts them to comply with the rules, regulations, and laws surrounding patient privacy standards
4. C. permission by the patient to use or disclose his/her health information
5. G. written patient permission to copy medical information
6. E. protection of data, information, and information networks from unauthorized use
7. B. unwritten patient consent that allows individuals involved in the patient's care and treatment access to personal medical information

Professional MT Ethics

I. TRUE/FALSE.

1. false
2. false
3. true
4. false
5. true

II. MULTIPLE CHOICE.

1. dignity
2. timely
3. implement
4. integrity
5. comply with